1001 Healthy Baby Answers

Pediatricians' Answers to All the Questions You Didn't Know to Ask

Gary C. Morchower, MD

With contributions from the pediatric specialists at Medical City Children's Hospital

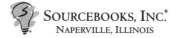
SOURCEBOOKS, INC.®
NAPERVILLE, ILLINOIS

Published by Sourcebooks, Inc.
P.O. Box 4410, Naperville, Illinois 60567–4410
(630) 961–3900
Fax: (630) 961–2168
www.sourcebooks.com

Library of Congress Cataloging-in-Publication Data

Morchower, Gary C.
   The healthy baby handbook : expert answers to all the questions you didn't know to ask / Gary C. Morchower.
      p. cm.
   1. Children—Diseases--Handbooks, manuals, etc. 2. Children--Health and hygiene—Handbooks, manuals, etc. I. Title.

RJ61.M7275 2008
618.92'02--dc22

                                        2007051004

Printed and bound in the United States of America.
BG 10 9 8 7 6 5 4 3 2 1

Dedication

To my children, Andrew and Karen, and to
my wife, Bette, the best mom of them all.

Acknowledgments

My sincere thanks to Lynda Pieper for her outstanding assistance in the electronic editing of this book.

Contents

Introduction

Definition:
A Message to Every Parent Who's Ever
Taken a Child to the Doctor

How many times have you returned with your child from the pediatrician's office, only to realize that you remember little of what was said to you during the visit? Perhaps it was because your mind was numb from staying up late taking care of your sick child, or possibly you were so worried about your child's illness that you could only focus on a few things that were discussed during the visit. Maybe you just accept that your doctor is knowledgeable, and the only issue of concern to you now is that your child gets better.

If any of these scenarios sound familiar, you are not alone. In my thirty-seven years of practice, I've seen medicine change dramatically, and that has impacted the type, length, and tenor of the pediatric office visit. Traditionally, families stayed with the same pediatrician throughout childhood, so they became comfortable with each other over the years. Now, with the emergence of managed care, families may change doctors as often as their employers change insurance plans. This can result in a game of "musical doctors," with the parent having to adapt to the styles, routines, and personalities of different doctors all too frequently.

Also, in the past, parents often relied on a helpful nurse to explain everything after the doctor left the room and to answer questions that came up. Now, nurses are just as busy as doctors, and it's less likely that you'll develop any better relationship with them, as you may see different nurses or nurse assistants at every office visit.

Perhaps the biggest change, though, is the length of the office visit. Doctors nowadays are more pressed for time than ever. Once they've established the appropriate diagnosis, they frequently deliver the treatment plan quickly, bombarding the parent with information. Consequently, the parent leaves the office with only a vague idea of what is going on.

Adding to the problem is that parents are often leery of questioning medical advice. Questions that should be asked often don't get asked. As a result, important areas of concern are not addressed—or worse, the treatment is misinterpreted or misunderstood.

Too often, I've heard parents say, "You mean he was supposed to finish the medicine even though he was feeling better?" or "I didn't know I was supposed to bring my daughter back for a follow-up" or "I thought I was to continue giving my child only clear liquids until the diarrhea had completely cleared." The consequences of these misunderstandings may be minimal in some cases, but other times the result is a recurrence of the original illness or the development of a complication.

I wrote this book because I don't want that to happen to your child. I want you to feel like you can ask your doctor questions even if you think they might seem silly. It's critical that you understand your child's condition fully and that you have all the information you need to help your child get better.

The book is organized into three parts. The first deals with conditions specific to newborns—those that show up at birth or in the hospital. The second consists of the most common conditions experienced by children and adolescents. Finally, there is a section on questions to ask when choosing a pediatrician. The book is organized alphabetically by disease, with a series of questions listed for each condition. You don't need to become a physician to help your child get better, you just need to know the right questions to ask.

In addition, there are reference answers listed for each question to supplement information obtained from your own pediatrician. The reference answers are supplied by the pediatric specialist physicians at Medical City Children's Hospital in Dallas, Texas. Each of these specialists is an expert in his or her own medical field. The answers provided are an excellent source of information to better understand your child's condition and how to manage it.

I hope you'll bring this book with you to every office visit. Use it after the doctor has given you the diagnosis and formal treatment plan. If you forget or get distracted, call back later, book in hand, and use the questions to fill in the blanks to your understanding. Take plenty of notes, so along with the specialist reference answers, you will have something to refer to when the memory of the doctor's verbal commentaries has faded.

How will your doctor feel about your newfound inquisitiveness? Many parents worry that questions such as these might irritate or alienate the doctor. I couldn't disagree more! *When it comes to caring for your sick child, you have every right to ask whatever questions you need to clarify what the illness is and how you should treat it.*

In reality, the questions in this book and the reference answers provided are meant to complement the office visit and will only enhance the effectiveness of what the doctor is trying to accomplish. Most pediatricians want parents to leave with as much knowledge about the child's illness as possible. Indeed, it is my sincere hope that this book will enhance the relationship between you and your child's doctor and that you have many productive and healthy visits down the road for years to come.

Contributing Specialists

ALLERGY AND IMMUNOLOGY
Elliot J. Ginchansky, MD
Robert W. Sugerman, MD
Richard L. Wasserman, MD

CARDIOLOGY
Jane Kao, MD
W. Pennock Laird, II, MD

CRANIOFACIAL SURGERY
Jeffrey A. Fearon, MD
David Genecov, MD

DERMATOLOGY
K. Robin Carder, MD

DEVELOPMENTAL PEDIATRICS
Lisa W. Genecov, MD

ENDOCRINOLOGY
Ellen S. Sher, MD

GASTROENTEROLOGY
Jack An, MD
Eric Argao, MD
Kendall O. Brown, MD
Annette Whitney, MD

GENETICS
Angela Scheuerle, MD

GYNECOLOGY
Kelli Watkins, MD

HEMATOLOGY
Carl Lenarsky, MD

INFECTIOUS DISEASES
Wendy Chung, MD
Stuart W. Ehrett, MD
Gregory R. Istre, MD

NEONATOLOGY
Clair Schwendeman, MD

NEPHROLOGY
Albert Quan, MD

NEUROLOGY
Roy D. Elterman, MD
Steven L. Linder, MD
David B. Owen, MD

OPHTHALMOLOGY
Joel Leffler, MD
David Stager, Jr, MD

ORTHOPEDICS
Roderick Capelo, MD
W. Barry Humeniuk, MD

OTOLARYNGOLOGY
(Ear, Nose, and Throat)
Paul W. Bauer, MD

Michael Biavati, MD
Timothy Trone, MD

PODIATRY
Donald Blum, DPM

PSYCHIATRY
Dante Burgos, MD

PULMONARY
Andrew S. Gelfand, MD
Peter N. Schochet, MD
Richard B. Silver, MD

SLEEP MEDICINE
Hilary Pearson, MD

SURGERY
Kevin M. Kadesky, MD
John L. LaNoue, MD

UROLOGY
Adam G. Baseman, MD
David Ewalt, MD
William Strand, MD

Part I

Common Conditions in Newborns

ARM PARALYSIS
(Brachial Plexus Palsy)

Definition: Paralysis or weakness of the arm muscles.

1. How did this condition occur in my baby?

Brachial plexus palsy is caused by a stretch injury of the nerves supplying the muscles of the upper extremity (brachial plexus) during delivery. Recognized risk factors include large birth weight, breech position, prolonged labor, difficult delivery, shoulder dystocia, and neonatal distress.

The causes of this stretch are due to the forces of labor, especially in cases of shoulder dystocia, and extraction maneuvers. Greater trauma occurs with forceful arm extraction maneuvers during a breech delivery. Exactly how much stretch is needed to produce permanent injury in any infant is not known.

2. Is my baby experiencing any discomfort?

No. This condition is caused by injury to the nerves supplying strength and sensation to the arm. Typical symptoms include asymmetric infantile reflexes and decreased spontaneous movement of the affected arm. If the child appears to be in pain, other conditions such as fractures of the clavicle (collarbone), humerus (upper arm bone), and shoulder should be ruled out with an X ray. Bone and/or joint infections should also be ruled out by blood tests, if pain is present.

3. What tests are needed to further define the condition?

X rays and blood tests may be required to rule out other conditions that can cause your child to have decreased movement of one extremity. Usually, no further tests are needed once the diagnosis has been made.

4. What is the treatment, and will physical therapy be needed?

Initial treatment includes protecting the involved limb by pinning the sleeve to the shirt or wrapping it to the body for the first several weeks. As soon as your child can tolerate it, gentle range of motion exercises should be started. These can typically be performed at home by the parents. Many infants will recover spontaneously on their own in the first six to eight weeks of life, and many will progress to a normal result. Those infants who do not initiate recovery until after three months of age may require future surgery to optimize the function of the arm.

5. How long will it take for the condition to be corrected, and will there be any residual weakness or decreased function of the arm?

If recovery is to occur on its own, it most commonly begins in the first six to eight weeks of life. If little or no active motion of the affected arm begins before three months of age, surgical procedures are commonly necessary to maintain motion of the shoulder, elbow, and wrist. Even after surgery, some residual decrease in function is very likely.

6. Should a neurologist or an orthopedist be consulted?

Consultation with an orthopedist should be initiated as soon as the diagnosis is made. Often, an orthopedist will assist in ruling out other conditions and in establishing the diagnosis in a newborn with decreased spontaneous movement of an arm.

7. When do you wish to see my baby again for this condition?

Your orthopedist will need to reassess the child every few weeks to ensure that the parents are performing the range of motion exercises properly and for signs of recovery. The decision whether to perform surgery or continue nonoperative treatment is usually made at three months of age.

RODERICK CAPELO, MD
Orthopedics

BIRTH DEFECT

Definition: **Any structural difference in the baby's body. Also called congenital anomaly or congenital malformation.**

1. What are birth defects?

Birth defects are changes in the normal structure of the body that are present when the baby is born. They may be minor problems, like a small extra finger or a large birthmark, or significant problems, such as a missing limb or an abnormal heart.

2. What causes birth defects?

Some birth defects are caused by genetic problems such as chromosome abnormalities or mutations (changes) in a particular gene. Other defects are caused by exposure to a toxin during pregnancy. Alcohol, the acne medicine isotretinoin (Accutane), and methyl mercury are recognized as causing birth defects if the fetus is exposed to these substances early in the pregnancy. Some birth defects are multifactorial; they have many factors that cause them, some of which are genetic and some of which are environmental.

3. What sort of tests should be done on my child?

The specific tests that your physician may perform will depend on what part of the body is affected. Typical tests include ultrasounds of the head and abdomen, X rays, CT or MRI scans, and echocardiograms (ultrasounds of the heart). These tests are done to determine how serious the problem is and whether there are other problems. Your child may get some or all of these tests.

Genetic testing is done to try to determine the cause of the birth defect. These may include an analysis of the baby's chromosomes, tests for specific mutations, or tests of the baby's metabolism.

4. What is the treatment for birth defects?

The treatment depends on the birth defect. Some do not need treatment. Some can be treated easily while the baby is in the nursery or soon after birth. Many require monitoring by a specialist, and some can only be fixed using surgery.

5. No one else in the family has this problem; why did it happen to my child?

About one out of every twenty babies (5 percent) are born with some sort of birth defect. There are many things that have to go right in order for babies to be born normal. Sometimes this just doesn't happen. Much of the time it is impossible to say why a particular baby has a birth defect. Sometimes a problem can run in a family without causing difficulty until a baby is born with a serious version of it.

6. Do we need to consult with a geneticist or any other specialist?

Yes. All babies with birth defects can benefit from seeing a doctor who specializes in genetics. The geneticist will help determine whether the problem is isolated or whether there is a larger "syndrome." It is always helpful to have the input of a geneticist before undergoing genetic testing. He or she can also help find out whether the problem runs in the family and what your chances are of having another affected child.

7. Will my next child have birth defects?

Whether birth defects will happen in another child depends on what the defects are and what caused them. All pregnancies have a risk of about 5 percent (one in twenty) that the baby will have a birth defect. Having one child with a birth defect increases your chances of having another. The first step is to have a firm diagnosis of the problem in your affected child.

8. How early can birth defects be diagnosed?

Large birth defects, such as spina bifida, can be detected in the late first trimester of pregnancy. As pregnancy progresses and the fetus gets larger, other birth defects can become apparent. If your doctor knows you have one child with a particular problem, then the doctor can specifically look for that problem. Some birth defects, such as cleft palate, are very difficult to diagnose before birth. All birth defects can be diagnosed after birth, but some are not found until the child is older, or unless they cause a problem.

9. Is there a way to prevent birth defects?

Every pregnancy is at risk for birth defects. There is no guaranteed way to eliminate all of them, but you can reduce the risk. Here are some ways to reduce your risk of having a child with birth defects:

- Be as healthy as possible *before* you get pregnant. Control chronic illnesses and start taking prenatal vitamins or at least folic acid supplements.
- Plan and space out your pregnancies and get good care during your pregnancy.
- Do not smoke or drink alcohol while pregnant. Do not use any medications without talking to your doctor. Remember that everything that you put in your body also is going into the baby's body.
- Seek out information about your personal risk from a geneticist if anyone in your family has a birth defect or has had a child who died or required surgery before one year of age. The same applies to someone who comes from a culture in which people marry within the extended family or someone who has had two or more pregnancy losses.

10. Will in vitro fertilization prevent birth defects?

No. There are some fertility treatments that can be used to avoid a particular birth defect or genetic condition, but there is never a guarantee that a child will be normal. It has also been found that artificial reproductive techniques have a higher than normal incidence of certain problems in the baby. One of these problems is hypospadias, which is an abnormality of the penis. Another problem is called an imprinting defect. This is an abnormality in the way the early embryo manages the genetic material that can lead to some specific genetic syndromes.

ANGELA SCHEUERLE, MD
Genetics

BLOOD INFECTION
(Bacterial Sepsis)

Definition: **A serious condition caused by multi-plying bacteria in the bloodstream.**

1. What caused this condition?

Infections due to bacteria in the bloodstream may occur during the birthing process when bacteria from the birth canal get onto the newborn's skin, nose, mouth, and eyes. These bacteria can then get into the lungs and/or bloodstream to cause the infection.

Another way that the newborn may become infected is by bacteria infecting the placenta and getting into the infant's bloodstream through the placenta and umbilical cord. The most common bacteria that cause neonatal infections are *Group B streptococcus*, *Listeria monocytogenes*, and *Escherichia coli* (*E. coli*). Occasionally, viruses such as *herpes* or *cytomegalovirus* may also cause infections in the newborn.

2. What problems does it pose?

Infections in newborns can be relatively minor, causing problems such as mild breathing issues, decreased temperature, or low blood sugar.

They can also be life-threatening or fatal, resulting in severe breathing concerns, decreased heart function, and/or seizures.

3. What tests are needed to further define the condition?

The growing of the bacteria or virus on a culture, which is a test performed by applying samples of the baby's blood onto a plate with nutrients, confirms the presence of an infection in the blood. In addition to blood, samples of the airway secretions; swabs of the eyes, nose, and skin; urine; and spinal fluid (spinal tap) may also be collected and tested in this manner.

4. How is blood infection treated?

Antibiotics are used to kill the bacteria causing the infection. Some viral infections can be treated with antiviral medications. The laboratory tests (culture) will confirm which medications are most effective in treating the infection. In serious infections, other medications and treatments may be necessary to assist with breathing, to help the heart function properly, and to control seizures.

5. Do we need to consult with a neonatologist (newborn specialist) or an infectious disease specialist?

Very minor or "suspected" infections can be treated by the pediatrician. If the infection is significant or other support is needed, then referral to a neonatologist and/or an infectious disease specialist should occur.

6. How long will it take for my baby to recover from this illness?

Infections that are confirmed in the bloodstream will require a minimum of seven to fourteen days treatment with intravenous (IV) antibiotics. If the infection is in the spinal fluid, the antibiotics may be required for up to twenty-one days or more. Depending on the seriousness of the infection, the time for recovery may extend beyond the end of taking antibiotics.

7. Will this condition weaken my baby in any way in the future, and will there be any long-term ill effects caused by it?

In serious infections or infections that involve the spinal fluid or the brain, there can be long-term effects, such as movement abnormalities, mental retardation, cerebral palsy, or hearing loss. There may be some continuing lung abnormalities due to the use of a breathing machine. Occasionally, the blood infection also infects a joint or bone. This could result in an injury to that joint or a limitation of the growth of the bone.

8. How long will my baby have to stay in the hospital as a result of this disorder?

At least seven to fourteen days will be required, as the antibiotics to treat the infection have to be given through an IV. In serious infections with complications it may be a month or longer.

9. After discharge from the hospital, what kind of follow-up will be needed?

Infections that did not require significant levels of support other than antibiotics may be monitored under routine care by the pediatrician. If there are complications, especially of the brain and nervous system, developmentalists or neurologists (specialists that monitor the development of the brain) may be recommended.

CLAIR SCHWENDEMAN, MD
Neonatology

CEPHALOHEMATOMA

Definition: A swelling of the scalp caused by a hemorrhage under the outer layer of bone in one area of the skull.

1. What caused this condition?

The swelling associated with this condition is a result of the scalp tissues being injured during the delivery process.

There are several types of swelling of the scalp that can occur, based on the depth of the swelling and/or the amount of bleeding involved. The different types of swelling are caput succedaneum, cephalohematoma, and subgaleal hematoma. Most types are more common with vaginal deliveries than cesarean sections.

Caput succedaneum: Superficial layers of the scalp with swelling and bruising that generally improves significantly prior to discharge from the hospital.

Cephalohematoma: Bleeding between the outer layer of the scalp bone and the lining of the bone. It is more contained and does not spread past the edge of the bone. It is often present along with caput

succedaneum. When the superficial swelling goes away, it is more identifiable. The affected areas are soft and may be on one or both sides of
the scalp. They may take several months to completely dissolve. As
they go away, they may have a crunchy or crackly feeling to them.

Subgaleal hematoma: Bleeding that occurs deeper under the skin
layers, but above the outer layer of the bones. This swelling can be
seen all around the scalp and may push the ears forward slightly. Due
to the amount of bleeding that can occur, it requires close monitoring
and occasionally blood transfusions.

2. Is it potentially dangerous?

Cephalohematomas and subgaleal hemorrhages can be potentially
dangerous depending on the amount of bleeding that occurs. Some
cephalohematomas can also include fractures of the skull and bleeding
inside the bones of the skull.

3. Does this condition represent any possible injury to the brain?

The majority of the time, there is no injury to the brain, as all the
bleeding is small and outside of the skull. Rarely, when there is bleeding
that occurs inside the skull, the brain may be at risk for injury.

4. What tests are needed to further define the condition?

The majority of the time, nothing needs to be done except a physical
examination and observation. When there are concerns for larger
amounts of bleeding, a blood count may be performed. In rare
instances of concern for a skull fracture or bleeding on the inside of
the skull, X rays of the skull and/or a CT scan of the skull and brain
may be performed.

5. Are there any other potential problems that can occur in the future?

In the first week of life, the baby may have to be watched more closely for jaundice that needs treatment. The risk for significant jaundice increases with the amount of bleeding and the destruction of the red blood cells within the swollen area. If there are fractures of the skull, most do not need treatment. Also, bleeding inside the skull generally does not need surgery unless it is progressive and causes excessive pressure on the brain.

6. Over what period of time can we expect this condition to improve?

Caputs generally improve within several days. Cephalohematomas may take up to six months to resolve.

7. How often will you need to see my baby for follow-up after discharge from the hospital?

In most cases there is no needed special follow-up for this swelling. If there are concerns about jaundice, a daily blood test may be needed for several days after discharge from the hospital. In severe cases where there are skull fractures or bleeding inside the skull, follow up with a neurosurgeon (surgeon of the brain) may be necessary.

CLAIR SCHWENDEMAN, MD
Neonatology

CHROMOSOMAL ABNORMALITIES

Definition: A type of genetic condition caused by large changes in genetic material. Most often found in children with multiple birth defects or complex problems starting from birth.

1. What are chromosomes?

Chromosomes are the structures in all the cells of our body that store our genetic information. They are large pieces of deoxyribonucleic acid (DNA). Human beings normally have forty-six chromosomes.

2. What features does my baby have that make you suspect this kind of disorder?

Your baby has physical features that are unusual for your family. These may be major differences, like missing eyes or an abnormal heart. Or the different features may be minor, like ears that are not in the right place or short fingers. The specific features vary depending on which chromosome is involved.

3. How did my baby develop this type of condition?

Most of the time, chromosome problems happen during formation of the egg or sperm. Sometimes a chromosomal rearrangement happens soon after conception in the early embryo. Rarely, the chromosome problem is inherited from a parent. When it is inherited, the parent may have a similar problem, or the parent may be unaffected.

4. What tests are needed to further define the disorder?

The most common test is a chromosome analysis, or karyotype. This is done using a blood sample. About a teaspoon of blood is collected and sent to a cytogenetics lab (the kind of lab that looks at chromosomes). The lab will process the sample, take pictures of the chromosomes, count them, and look at them closely. The lab is looking for large changes in the chromosomes, such as a missing or extra piece. This type of test does not see small changes in the genetic material. The chromosome analysis takes ten days to two weeks.

Fluorescence in situ hybridization (FISH) is a way of looking at smaller pieces of genetic material. Depending upon your baby's specific features, a FISH test may be ordered. A newer type of test is the Chromosome Microarray Analysis (CMA), which can also test for changes in smaller pieces of genetic material. It may be ordered rather than a FISH test.

5. What kind of impairments can occur as a result of this condition?

If your baby has a physical abnormality, like a missing hand or foot, there will be impairments because of that. Most chromosome abnormalities cause some amount of mental retardation. The retardation can be severe. Large chromosome abnormalities, which involve significant changes in the genetic material, can cause death in infancy or childhood.

6. Is this disorder treatable?

There is no cure for chromosome problems. There is no way to take out the abnormal chromosome and put in a normal one. However, your child will get whatever treatment is needed. Treatment may include physical therapy or heart surgery and will be determined by the specific needs of your child.

7. Is it possible that any of our future children might be born with this disorder?

When a baby has a chromosome problem, it is typical to test both parents. If the parents both have normal chromosomes, the risk of giving birth to another affected child is not increased; the risk is the same as it is for anyone. (There is never zero risk.) If one parent has a chromosome abnormality, the chance of having another child affected with a chromosome problem is at least fifty-fifty. Depending upon what the chromosome problem is, the chance of having an affected child may be as high as two out of three.

8. Do we need to consult with a geneticist or any other specialist?

Yes. Your baby should be seen by a doctor who specializes in genetics. The geneticist can help get testing done and talk to you about what to expect from your child. The geneticist can also discuss your chances of having other affectecd children and may be able to put you in touch with other families who have children with the same problem.

9. What kind of special plans should be made to care for the baby once we arrive home?

Your baby will need all the routine pediatric care, including immunizations. If your baby has special health needs, like tube feedings, you should be taught about that at the hospital. Sometimes babies with chromosome problems are not expected to live very long. You may choose to enroll your baby in a hospice program. Hospice programs support you and the baby so that the family can have a good quality of life, even if your baby's time within the family is short.

10. When do you wish to see my baby again for this condition?

It is likely that your baby will have many different doctors. There will also be occupational and physical therapy, and your baby may need surgery. Your pediatrician can help coordinate all the different doctors.

ANGELA SCHEUERLE, MD
Genetics

CLEFT LIP/CLEFT PALATE

Definition: A birth defect consisting of a cleft deformity of the lip and/or the palate.

Author's Comment: Fortunately, the medical repair of this type of
birth defect, which can appear so intimidating at birth, is amazingly
good and far superior to the cosmetic corrections of the past.

1. What caused this condition to occur in my child?

The condition is due to multiple factors. Cleft lip with or without
a cleft palate can be an inherited condition, but more commonly is
the result of a developmental break in the fusion of the facial
segments. Exposure to heavy metals, deficiencies of vitamin B12
and folate, and environmental factors can all play a part in causing
these deformities. The condition can be associated with more
complex facial syndromes but is less common than singular presen-
tation alone.

2. Did something I did or did not do during my pregnancy contribute to the cause?

Expectant mothers who do not take prenatal vitamins and do not receive prenatal care are associated with a higher increase in complications in the newborn period as well as structural deformities at birth (congenital anomalies). However, because cleft lip/cleft palate is such a complex anomaly, it is very difficult to pinpoint the cause or directly relate causation to something the mother did or did not do.

3. When do we need to see a plastic surgeon that specializes in the repair of this type of problem (craniofacial surgeon)? Will the surgeon show me pictures of children with this deformity who have had the repair procedure(s)?

When the diagnosis is made, often based on a prenatal ultrasound, the parents should seek the advice and consultation of a craniofacial/cleft surgeon. This allows the family to be prepared for the delivery and to get most of their questions answered prior to the hustle and bustle of the postnatal period.

The surgeon should see the infant at two weeks' discharge from the hospital for a complete examination to evaluate the presence of other problems. A surgeon should be able to show before and after pictures of surgeries he or she has performed. Additionally, many practices can get you in touch with parents of other children with cleft lip and/or palate deformities so that you can get the information you need on a parent-to-parent basis.

4. What kind of surgery or reconstruction procedure(s) will be needed to repair this deformity, and when will they occur?

Children with cleft lip and/or palate deformities often undergo a series of operations within the first two years of life. This usually first includes a lip repair (possibly with a nasal correction at the same time) at around three months of age. The surgery can be delayed if the child is born prematurely or is of slight stature. The child should be at least ten weeks old, weigh 10 pounds, and have a hemoglobin (measurement of the blood count) level of 10 before undergoing this surgery.

The palate is then repaired between six to twelve months of age depending on the surgeon. Many surgeons repair the palate in one stage at or near twelve months of age to promote good speech.

Each surgeon should have a protocol that works for him or her and is specific to each center. It is recommended that you seek a surgeon associated with a respected and affiliated center so that the child can receive complete care from team of specialists, including a speech pathologist, pediatric dentist, geneticist, pediatric anesthesiologist, and pediatric ear, nose, and throat specialist. These people will be closely integrated into the child's care.

After the first year, there can be additional operations depending on the severity of the cleft and the resulting facial changes during growth. Many issues present themselves over time as the child grows. The face often becomes asymmetric and deficient on the cleft side. Operations can include a bone graft into the cleft at the level of the gum line, a nasal procedure to improve breathing and straighten the nose, and even jaw surgery to improve the bite and facial balance. Further surgeries are performed on an individual basis. The goal is to keep the child's facial features as symmetric and functional as possible throughout growth.

5. What are the dangers of the surgery?

Surgery on children carries the same or similar dangers as surgery on adults, such as bleeding, infection, scarring, and persistence of the asymmetries. Other issues include persistent holes in the palate (fistulas) and palatal dysfunction that may lead to speech impediments, most specifically a nasal voice or inadequate functioning of the soft palate and the upper part of the throat (velopharyngeal insufficiency).

Many dangers are unpredictable because they depend on the age of the child and the level of the original deformity. As with other conditions, life-threatening risks are associated with any surgery and are closely related to anesthesia. Therefore, it is important to have an anesthesiologist specially trained in the care of children to do the surgical cases.

6. How will the deformity impact my child's functioning, and what can be done to overcome it?

In children with cleft lip and palate deformities, the scars are often visible. The impact of this deformity is hard to address. Of course, the child will be aware of his or her differences from other children, and this awareness usually begins between the ages of two and four years old. I tell all of my patients that we all have scars of some form. Addressing the scars directly helps the child deal with these differences better. Consistent parent and family support, open dialogue as the child gets older, and the child's inclusion in surgical and care decisions as he or she is able all help diminish the negative effects of the congenital deformity.

7. Is there a greater likelihood that my child will have more learning differences or speech problems than other children?

Children with cleft lip (but not cleft palate) have no greater incidence of speech or learning differences than other children. However, when the palate is involved, the risk of speech issues significantly increases. These children should be followed yearly, if not more frequently, for speech issues throughout their growth.

In 10 percent to 15 percent of cases, children with a cleft palate may require further surgery to improve their speech. As far as learning differences go, it is hard to tell the likelihood that they will occur, as there is not much data available in this area. Since children with cleft palate also have a higher incidence of hearing problems, it is these hearing issues that can lead to learning difficulties because the child cannot always hear what is going on in the classroom. Once fixed, these issues resolve.

8. If we have future children, what are the chances that they will be born with this same type of disorder?

The incidence of having a child with a cleft lip/palate deformity is about one in seven hundred. If either parent or a first-degree family member has the deformity, the risk increases. If you have one child with the deformity, the risk of subsequent children having a clefting deformity also increases. Because of these increased risks, genetic counseling is recommended prior to having further children so parents can have a complete understanding of these risks.

9. What kind of follow-up will be needed for this condition?

Children with cleft lip and palate deformities require consistent follow-up with the cleft palate team throughout their growth, which is usually until their high school graduation. Because there are changes during growth, the final effects of the deformity are not seen until growth is complete. Different stages of a child's development require different surgical, orthodontic, and therapeutic interventions.

Each member of the team may need to see the child independently, but the entire team should follow up yearly. It is key that the child is cared for by a team of physicians and health care specialists who are trained specifically in the care of the cleft patient, as this regimen of close follow-up is mandatory.

DAVID GENECOV, MD
Craniofacial Surgery

CLUBFOOT

Definition: **A type of structural deformity of the foot present at birth.**

1. What caused this condition to occur?

"Clubfoot" is a term that describes a complex, abnormal structural alignment of the bones and joints of the foot and ankle. It most likely represents abnormal development of many tissue types below the knee. The exact cause of clubfoot is still debated. It is likely caused by multiple factors, including genetic and environmental factors. Proposed theories of the cause of clubfoot include molding of the foot while still in the womb (*in utero* molding), primary muscle problems, primary bone deformity, primary blood vessel lesion, intrauterine viral infection, primary nerve lesion, and abnormal stiffening of the tissues. The actual cause is likely a combination of these factors.

2. What exactly is structurally wrong with the foot?

The appearance of clubfeet are created by both the malalignment of the bones at the joints and the altered shape of the bones. In addition, the muscles, ligaments, tendons, and connective tissue (fascia) of the foot and ankle are contracted, or shortened. The result is a rigid foot that is turned downward and inward.

3. How is it treated, and how successful is the treatment?

The goal of treatment is a painless, flexible foot that strikes the ground in proper position when walking. Regardless of the severity or rigidity, the initial treatment is nonoperative, using repeated sequential castings, also called "serial castings." The goal of this kind of treatment is to limit the amount of surgery required.

Nonoperative treatment involves weekly serial castings to promote gradual correction of the foot over six to eight weeks. Following this casting regimen, nearly all children require a short outpatient surgical procedure to fully correct the foot. Then a special brace is worn full time for eight to nine months and part time for two to three years.

The ability to completely correct the clubfoot deformity depends on each child's unique initial severity and rigidity, the age at which treatment is started, the skill of the orthopedic surgeon, and the definition of complete correction. Although the position of the foot may be dramatically improved with treatment, nearly all patients with clubfoot have a difference in calf size, foot size, and possibly overall limb length compared to unaffected limbs. Eighty percent of children have a painless functional foot following serial manipulation and casting.

4. Will my child be able to walk and exercise normally following treatment?

Most children who undergo successful nonoperative treatment are able to walk normally. Because this is an abnormality of most of the tissues below the knee, some difference between normal limbs will always be observed. In a fully corrected foot, light exercise is generally well tolerated.

5. Do you think that there will be any limitations or disadvantages athletically because of this condition?

Again, the goal of nonoperative treatment is a painless, supple, properly positioned foot. Generally, there is some residual stiffness and weakness compared to normal limbs. Depending on the initial severity and degree of correction achieved and maintained, there will likely be some degree of limitation athletically.

6. When do we need to see an orthopedic surgeon?

Consultation with a pediatric orthopedic surgeon should take place when the diagnosis is made. Serial manipulation and casting should be initiated as early as possible, preferably within the first week of life.

7. After discharge from the hospital, what kind of follow-up will be needed for this condition?

If consultation with your pediatric orthopedic surgeon did not occur prior to discharge from the hospital, your child should be seen in the office in the first week of life. Weekly follow-up visits for manipulation and casting will be necessary for the first six to eight weeks. Periodic follow-up will be necessary throughout childhood.

RODERICK CAPELO, MD
Orthopedics

HEART DISEASE–CONGENITAL

Definition: Abnormalities of the heart or conduction system that occur at birth.

1. What is wrong with my baby's heart, and what problems does the defect cause?

A congenital heart defect is a birth defect of the heart. Many different types of defects exist. The most common type of defect is a hole in either the upper or lower wall of the heart. Both of these defects result in an excess amount of blood flow to the lungs. Other defects include abnormalities with the heart valves, resulting in the heart muscle having to work harder than normal to pump blood to the lungs or body.

2. Is the condition potentially dangerous?

Many congenital heart defects are minor and present no significant risk whatsoever to the child. However, some types of defects can be dangerous or even life threatening.

3. What tests are needed to further define the condition?

The most common test is an echocardiogram. This test uses sound waves to visualize the structures of the heart. In almost all cases, a clear diagnosis can be made based on the findings of an echocardiogram. Other tests that are often performed include pulse oximetry (checking the oxygen level in the blood), electrocardiography (assessing the heart's electricity), and a chest X ray to visualize both the heart and lungs.

4. Will my baby need surgery, and is the condition correctable?

The majority of congenital heart defects are minor in nature and require no specific treatment whatsoever. More serious defects may require surgery. Fortunately, in this day and age almost all congenital heart defects are correctable with surgery and have excellent outcomes.

5. Will any heart medicines be needed to treat this problem?

Most minor congenital heart defects do not require any medications whatsoever. More significant defects may require medications. Typically, medicine is used either to improve the pumping function of the heart or to relieve the lungs of any excess fluid.

6. Do we need to see a pediatric cardiologist and, if so, when?

Your pediatrician will determine whether it is necessary to see a pediatric cardiologist. Some types of minor congenital heart disease may not require a referral to a specialist. However, if a more significant heart defect is suspected, usually a referral is made at that time.

7. Will my baby become blue (cyanotic) from this condition?

Certain types of heart defects result in a blue appearance to the skin, termed cyanosis. This blue appearance results from an inadequate amount of oxygen in the blood, usually due to the blood failing to pass from the heart to the lungs. Blood with a normal amount of oxygen has a red or pink appearance to it, but blood lacking oxygen is blue. In general, heart defects resulting in cyanosis are fairly unusual and are usually noticed at or shortly after birth.

8. After I leave the hospital, what danger signs do I look for that would indicate that my baby is having a problem related to this condition?

Rapid breathing is one sign that might indicate a potential heart problem in a baby. This is usually caused by excessive blood flow to the lungs, although occasionally it may be due to a lower than normal oxygen level in the bloodstream. Other signs that might indicate a potential heart problem in a baby would include unusual color changes, such as a bluish or pale appearance to the skin, poor appetite, or unusual irritability.

9. Do I need to limit my baby's activities in any way after we go home?

Most babies diagnosed with heart problems do not need any limitation on their activities whatsoever. However, check with your doctor as the recommendation may vary based on the seriousness of your child's heart condition.

10.   After discharge from the hospital, when do you wish to see my baby again concerning this condition?

Usually, follow-up will be determined by the type of heart condition that your baby has been diagnosed with. Minor heart defects may only require reassessment at routine visits. More significant heart conditions may require more frequent checkups.

W. PENNOCK LAIRD, II, MD
Cardiology

HYPOGLYCEMIA

Definition: Low blood sugar.

1. What caused this condition to occur?

Hypoglycemia occurs when the baby's blood sugar (glucose) is low, with a measure that is less than 40 mg/dL to 45 mg/dL. Low blood sugar is due to a disruption or abnormality in the baby's blood sugar regulatory system and is most common in the first two hours after birth. Much of the time, it is corrected with early feeding and continued monitoring for the first twenty-four hours.

Babies born to mothers with diabetes or babies that are large for their age may have a more significant decrease in the blood sugar levels and need monitoring of the blood sugar level for several days. In rare cases, severe and quite prolonged low–blood sugar levels may require surgery, special diet, and/or medication.

2. Is hypoglycemia dangerous, and will it have any permanent impact on my baby's health?

In the majority of cases, when brief and treated promptly, there are no permanent effects of low blood sugar on the baby. However, untreated or prolonged blood sugar levels may lead to brain injury.

3. What tests are needed to further define the condition?

In most cases, a simple measurement of the blood sugar level by a machine at the bedside is all that is necessary. Sometimes a confirmation of the low measurement by the bedside machine will need to be performed. This is done by collecting a small amount of blood from the baby and sending it to the laboratory. In the rarer cases of severe and prolonged low blood sugar, blood levels of various hormones may be needed and may take several days to return.

4. How are we going to treat it, and are there any side effects that might occur from the treatments?

In most cases, the low blood sugar level is treated with either feedings alone or in combination with intravenous (IV) sugar solutions. Infrequently in more severe cases, medications may be also given either as an IV or by mouth. There are generally no side effects.

5. How long will the condition take to correct?

In infants that are born to mothers without diabetes and are normal size for their age, normal blood sugar levels will generally be obtained within three to six hours of birth and monitoring may continue for up to twenty-four hours. In infants that are born to mothers with diabetes or are large for their age, the ability to maintain normal blood sugar levels without treatment and monitoring may take three to five days or longer.

6. Is there a chance the condition might come back following discharge from the hospital, and is there any special need for follow-up?

As long as the baby is feeding normally, the vast majority of babies will not have any recurrence of low blood sugar, and no special follow-up is needed. In the rare cases of severe and prolonged low blood sugars where surgery, medications, and/or a special diet has been required, those infants will need continued monitoring at home and follow-up with pediatric endocrinologists, doctors that specialize in disorders of hormone levels or metabolism.

7. Does hypoglycemia predispose my baby to developing diabetes or any other sugar metabolism disorder later in life?

Infants born to long-standing diabetic mothers may have a genetic predisposition to developing diabetes. Infants born to mothers with high blood sugars during the pregnancy or mothers with later onset diabetes are not at an increased risk for developing diabetes later in life, but may be at higher risk to be obese in the preteen and teenage years.

8. Will future babies that I might have be more inclined to have hypoglycemia? Is there any precaution that I can take to prevent it from happening again?

Mothers that have high blood sugars or diabetes, either when not pregnant or just when pregnant, will continue to have infants that are at higher risk for low blood sugars after birth. Monitoring of blood sugars during pregnancy as needed and maintaining good control of the blood sugar levels prior to and during the pregnancy will decrease the risk of the infant.

9. After discharge from the hospital, when do you wish to see my baby again for this condition?

In the large majority of babies, there is no need for special follow-up. Babies should have demonstrated that they can maintain normal blood sugar levels for a period of time prior to discharge and are expected to continue to do so.

CLAIR SCHWENDEMAN, MD
Neonatology

HYPOSPADIAS

Definition: When the opening normally at the end of
the penis is located on the undersurface
of the penis.

1. What caused this condition to occur?

There are multiple possible causes with genetic, environmental, and
hormonal factors influencing development of the penis. No one is
certain as to the exact cause of this condition. The incidence of
hypospadias has been increasing worldwide over the past few decades.
The incidence is approaching 1 percent of newborns.

2. What tests need to be done to further define the condition?

Typically, the diagnosis is made on physical examination of the newborn.
The majority of boys with hypospadias will need no further evaluation to
help plan a treatment course. If your child has an undescended testicle
along with hypospadias, blood testing to evaluate for an endocrine
problem or other developmental conditions should be performed. Some

cases of severe hypospadias may also require such testing. It is not recommended to perform newborn circumcision in patients with hypospadias as the foreskin may be useful in reconstruction at a later date.

3. What kind of symptoms or problems can occur as a result of the condition?

The penis has basically two functions: urination and sex. Children with uncorrected hypospadias may be impacted in either or both of these categories. Penile curvature (chordee) associated with hypospadias may make penetration painful or difficult to achieve. Depending on the location of the urethral opening, urinating while standing may be impossible to perform without significant spraying and deflection of the urine stream. If the hypospadia is corrected, there should be no future problems in either area.

4. Will it need to be corrected? If so, when and how?

Almost all cases of hypospadias require surgical treatment, although some of the most minor hypospadias may not require any intervention. Many pediatric urologists will recommend surgery to be performed after four months of age.

There are over two hundred described techniques that are used for hypospadia repairs. Your physician will discuss the technique that will be best suited for your son's particular anatomy. There has been much advancement in technique over the past years, and now hypospadia repair is almost always done as a day surgery on an outpatient basis.

5. Do we need to see a urologist and, if so, when?

The timing of urologic consultation is up to you and your pediatrician. Hospital consultation may be warranted if there are concerns or uncertainty about the diagnosis. Otherwise, outpatient consultation is completely appropriate and can be performed anytime between zero and two months of age.

6. Is there a possibility that there will be a problem later on in sexual or urinary function?

As discussed above in question #3, there can be impact on both sexual or urinary function in patients with hypospadias. If the problem is corrected early in life, it is unlikely that there will be any future issues in either of these areas.

7. When do you wish to see my child again for this condition?

After the initial consultation with your urologist, either scheduling for correction or a follow-up visit for your child at around two months of age may be recommended. This will be influenced by the degree of hypospadias and any other medical issues that your child may have.

ADAM G. BASEMAN, MD
Urology

INTESTINAL INFLAMMATION
(Necrotizing Enterocolitis)

Definition: An acute inflammation of the inner lining of the bowel with the presence of membrane-like areas and superficial ulcerations. Also called NEC.

1. What caused this condition?

In most cases, the baby was born early or premature and has been given some type of feeding. The lining or barrier of the intestinal tract has been injured, and this injury has allowed bacteria to get into the wall of the intestine. The bacteria cause an infection, injury, or weakness to the intestinal wall and an inflammatory reaction in those areas.

2. What tests need to be done to further define the condition?

The confirmatory signs of necrotizing enterocolitis (NEC) are seen on X rays of the abdomen. When NEC is suspected, a culture (test for bacteria in the bloodstream), a complete blood count (CBC), and a test to determine the level of inflammation (CRP) may also be performed on the infant's blood. A series of X rays of the abdomen and blood are done for several days to monitor this condition. A consultation with a pediatric surgeon may also be requested.

3. What potential dangers does NEC pose?

NEC is a serious concern and will cause some setback in the baby's condition. There are "mild" causes of NEC involving a limited portion of the intestine that improve in twenty-four to forty-eight hours of starting treatment. There are other cases of NEC that involve extensive areas or all of the intestine and are progressive. These cases require surgery with possible removal of intestine and are life threatening. When all of the intestine is involved, there may be no treatment possible, and it is then a fatal condition.

4. What is the treatment for NEC, and how long will it take for my baby to recover?

The treatment for NEC is stopping any feedings, starting antibiotic therapy, administering medications to stabilize the blood pressure and blood components (e.g., platelets and plasma) to prevent bleeding, and supporting breathing. Often a pediatric surgeon will be requested to evaluate the baby. Monitoring with repeat X rays of the abdomen, blood testing, and physical examinations are performed, often as frequently as every six hours.

A surgery is needed if a hole (perforation) occurs in the intestine or if the baby is not getting better. If surgery is performed, frequently a section or sections of intestine may be removed and the ends of the intestine brought up to and through the abdominal wall. The surgeon may decide to place a piece of rubber drain in the abdominal space if the infant is unstable and will not tolerate a major operation.

The length of recovery may vary from ten to fourteen days in the cases that respond to medicines, to a prolonged (years long) dependence on IV fluids in cases where there has been extensive involvement or removal of intestine.

5. Are there any potential side effects of the treatment?

There are many side effects that are related to the infection and inflammation from the NEC. Several of the antibiotics used to treat the infection require blood levels to be monitored and may result in some hearing loss if too high (due to toxic effects of the antibiotics on the nerve function within the inner ear). Breathing failure, kidney failure, low blood pressure, and bleeding problems are common issues that occur with NEC. When needed, surgery may be performed in a less than stable situation. Blood and fluid losses due to bleeding abnormalities and inflammation may further worsen the situation. Decreased blood pressure and flow could also cause injury to the brain.

The baby may need prolonged IV nutrition, which could lead to liver injury, a need for stable IV access, and subsequent infections of the bloodstream. A complication that may occur four to six weeks after the infant recovers is a narrowing in the intestine that requires surgery to correct.

6. Is it possible that this condition could get worse?

When NEC is first suspected or diagnosed, it is difficult to predict if it will respond or progress despite adequate treatment. Close observation of the baby is needed in the first twenty-four to forty-eight hours after beginning treatment. Often the condition does get more serious before improving.

7. Do we need to consult a neonatologist (newborn specialist) or gastroenterologist (specialist of the digestive system)?

Neonatologists should be consulted and assist in or assume the care of a baby with NEC or suspected NEC. A pediatric surgeon is often consulted as well. A gastroenterologist is generally not required during the critical period and may become involved after recovery if the baby is not able to grow on feedings or if concerns of liver injury from long-term IV nutritional support is present.

8. Will I be able to breastfeed my baby during this illness?

No. The stoppage of any feeding, breast or formula, takes place when NEC is suspected or confirmed. Resting of the intestinal tract and antibiotics are the main therapies for NEC. The baby may not be able to feed for a minimum of seven days in suspected NEC. If NEC is confirmed, a minimum of ten to fourteen days is required.

9. After discharge from the hospital, what kind of follow-up will be needed?

If a narrowing in the intestinal tract is suspected or if there is evidence of an intestinal blockage, an X ray test with dye and consultation with a surgeon will be necessary. If there are continued issues regarding how well the infant is able to digest and absorb feedings or if the infant is sent home on IV nutrition, then a gastroenterologist may be necessary. Attention to developmental issues is also important.

CLAIR SCHWENDEMAN, MD
Neonatology

JAUNDICE

Definition: Yellow appearance of the skin caused by bile pigment deposits in the skin.

1. What is jaundice, and what caused it to appear in my baby?

Jaundice is a common condition occurring in newborn babies. It is a yellowish skin discoloration caused by a waste product in the body called bilirubin. Bilirubin is produced when certain proteins and red blood cells are destroyed, which is a normal process that happens early on after birth. Newborns are more likely to be jaundiced due to increased destruction of red blood cells and the body's slow processing of bilirubin due to an immature functioning liver.

2. Is jaundice dangerous?

In the majority of cases, jaundice is not a life-threatening or serious condition. The bilirubin levels can get high enough that treatment is needed. In most cases the treatment is relatively simple with special lights (see question #5).

If the bilirubin level gets to a serious level, then an exchange of the baby's blood (exchange transfusion) may be necessary. Fortunately, this is a rare occurrence.

3. What tests are needed to further define the condition?

Most of the time, a meter will first be placed to the baby's forehead as a screening test. If the meter level is elevated, then it will be necessary to do a blood test to measure the bilirubin level. A test for the blood type of the infant is generally necessary to determine if it is compatible with the mother's blood type, but most of the time this is done on blood from the umbilical cord at the time of delivery. If there is a concern about rapid destruction of the red blood cells, a blood count may be necessary.

4. What is considered to be a danger point for the bilirubin level?

The actual level that treatment is started is dependent on the baby's age at birth, the number of days since birth, and whether or not there are conditions causing increased and more rapid red blood cell destruction. If the bilirubin level is rising quickly or approaching 20 mg/dL or more, therapy is generally started. Levels above 25 mg/dL have been associated with deposits of bilirubin (staining) on portions of the brain in some babies. This staining can lead to brain damage and lifelong injury.

5. If my baby's bilirubin level exceeds the danger point, what kind of therapy will be given and will it correct the problem?

The main therapy is phototherapy. The baby is given eye protection and is placed with minimal clothing under special blue lights. These lights help in the removal of bilirubin. Phototherapy usually lasts from two to five days.

If the baby is dehydrated, IV fluids may be started to correct the dehydration. Sometimes, breast-feeding and breast milk may not be given while the baby is under treatment for the jaundice.

6. Is phototherapy safe, and will there be any bad consequences afterward?

Phototherapy with appropriate eye protection has no serious side effects. Sometimes babies pass more stools while under phototherapy. Also since they are uncovered, some will require a heating source to prevent them from getting cold.

7. How often do we follow the bilirubin level, and will we continue to follow the level at home following discharge from the hospital?

If there are concerns, the bilirubin level is generally followed daily. This continues until the bilirubin level stabilizes or starts to drop. There may be a need for ongoing blood levels after discharge as the jaundice can persist for the first several weeks.

8. Can my baby become anemic from this disorder?

No, not from the jaundice itself. Jaundice is more severe in babies when there is a process that causes rapid or increased destruction of the red blood cells. There may be an incompatibility between the blood types of mother and baby, a defect in the red blood cells, or excessive bleeding or bruising that could cause the anemia and also make the baby more likely to have jaundice that requires treatment.

9. Is there anything else we need to know concerning this condition and its management?

Bilirubin is mainly passed from the body in the stool. Good feedings and ensuring good hydration in the first two to four days of life can decrease the risk of significant jaundice.

Very high levels of jaundice can lead to a condition called kernicterus. This is when parts of the brain are stained by the bilirubin. Kernicterus leads to cerebral palsy and lifelong abnormalities of the nervous system.

10. After discharge from the hospital, what kind of follow-up will be needed?

As discussed earlier, some babies require continued monitoring of the blood levels after discharge. This may be daily for several days. Some babies may require readmission to the hospital for treatment with phototherapy. Your pediatrician will instruct you on the frequency for the blood tests on discharge from the hospital.

CLAIR SCHWENDEMAN, MD
Neonatology

KIDNEY ENLARGEMENT
(Hydronephrosis)

Definition: Swelling of the kidney as a result of
obstruction to the flow of urine.

1. What caused this condition?

Hydronephrosis in most babies is a minor condition that goes away on
its own. It likely represents increased urine production by the fetus
prior to delivery that goes away with time.

Occasionally, hydronephrosis may be due to an obstruction that is caused
by abnormal development of the ureter (the tube that carries the urine from
the kidney to the bladder). Hydronephrosis may also represent the backwash
of urine from the bladder to the kidney known as vesicoureteral reflux.

2. What tests are needed to further define the disorder?

In most cases, ultrasound imaging is used to discover kidneys that are
hydronephrotic. Once a kidney has been determined to be
hydronephrotic, depending on the age and gender of the baby, a bladder
X ray should be performed to look for backwash of urine up to the kidney

(vesicoureteral reflux) or blockage in the urethra if the child is male.

In other instances where the condition is quite severe, a nuclear medicine renal scan should be performed to rule out obstruction of the kidney. An obstruction might require surgical intervention to preserve the kidney.

If the hydronephrosis involves both kidneys, then further evaluation with a standard blood test should be performed in the hospital or office to make sure that kidney function is normal.

3. Is this condition causing my baby any pain or discomfort?

If the kidney is significantly swollen (dilated) or it is obstructed, the baby may have pain, nausea or vomiting, or even blood in the urine. However, most degrees of hydronephrosis do not cause any pain or discomfort.

4. Is it correctable, and will surgery be necessary?

Most hydronephrosis is minor and will resolve or improve on its own as the baby gets bigger. However, if the dilation is significant or severe, then this may represent an obstruction of the kidney that will require surgery to resolve the obstruction. If the dilation of the kidney is related to vesicoureteral reflux, and if the reflux does not resolve as the baby gets older, then correction of the reflux may be necessary. Blockage of the male urethra must be corrected with surgery.

5. Will it predispose my baby to kidney disease or infection in the future?

Most hydronephrosis does not predispose the kidney to disease or infection; however, if the dilation is related to vesicoureteral reflux, reflux is a risk factor for developing both bladder and kidney infections. If the dilation is severe and involves both kidneys, then kidney disease is a possibility.

6. Do we need to consult a urologist and, if so, when?

Once the diagnosis of hydronephrosis is made, the urologist should be consulted to review the X rays, perform a complete history and physical examination of the baby and then determine if any other further studies are necessary. While this is generally not an urgent condition, if the child is having pain, significant infections, or it involves both kidneys, then the urologist should see the child immediately.

7. How will the condition be monitored following discharge from the hospital, and what tests will need to be done?

An ultrasound and further studies are usually recommended approximately four to six weeks following discharge. Depending on whether or not the hydronephrosis is severe, a renal scan may need to be performed. If the hydronephrosis involves both kidneys, then a standard blood test would need to be performed to determine kidney function. If the child has not had an evaluation for vesicoureteral reflux, then a bladder X ray test would be necessary.

8. What danger signs should we look for after leaving the hospital that would indicate that the kidney problem might be getting worse?

The most common symptoms associated with severe hydronephrosis or an obstructed kidney is abdominal, side, or back pain and vomiting. Fever may represent a urinary infection.

9. After discharge from the hospital, when do you wish to see my baby again?

After the child is discharged, we will normally see the child back in our office for an ultrasound and further studies approximately four to six weeks later. See question #7 for details.

DAVID EWALT, MD
Urology

LUNG RUPTURE
(Pneumothorax or
Pneumomediastinum)

Definition: Free air in the chest cavity.

1. What has caused this condition?

There was a tear or rupture in the air sacs (alveoli) in the lungs. This tear allowed air to escape out of the lung and into either the space between the lung and the chest wall (pneumothorax) or into the tissues along the blood vessels (pneumomediastinum).

Pneumothorax is relatively common in newborn babies, occurring in approximately 1 percent of all newborns.

Many babies have no symptoms. Others have symptoms related to the compression of the lung(s) by the leaked air and need treatment and/or supplemental oxygen. Babies that have other breathing problems and require breath assistance from a breathing machine are at potentially higher risks to develop air leaks in their lungs.

2. How is it treated?

In a lot of cases when the baby is otherwise healthy and without symptoms, observation is all that is needed and the tear will heal itself and the air be reabsorbed. In cases where the air leak is larger and the baby is having symptoms, the air may need to be pulled out (aspirated) by putting a needle in the baby's chest wall.

After the air in the chest cavity is pulled out, the needle is removed, and the baby is monitored for recurrence. If the leak continues or if the baby is on a breathing machine for support, a drainage tube (chest tube) is placed in the chest wall to continuously drain the air until the leak heals.

Many babies that have symptoms due to the free air will also require extra oxygen to keep their oxygen levels in an acceptable range. During this time, your baby may be breathing faster than normal or harder than normal and not be able to feed by mouth. This may require feedings via a tube, or the feedings withheld and IV fluids started.

3. How long will it take to correct itself?

This depends on the size of the leak. Many babies with small leaks that seal over rapidly are better in twelve to twenty-four hours, sometimes without symptoms. Babies that require needle aspiration or drainage tube placement may require two to three days or more to close the tear and allow the lungs to heal.

4. Do we need to consult with a neonatologist (newborn specialist) or a pediatric surgeon?

If the baby has symptoms or requires aspiration, drainage tube placement, or extra oxygen, a neonatologist is often involved in the care. Babies that are just breathing a bit fast or have no symptoms are often watched in newborn nursery by the pediatrician. It is rare that a surgeon or surgery is needed.

5. What tests need to be done to further define the condition?

An X ray of the chest is the test that absolutely confirms that a pneumothorax or pneumomediastinum is present. It can also provide some information as to how much air and compression on the lungs has occurred. Prior to the chest X ray, you may be able to suspect an air leak by listening to the chest and hearing decreased breath sounds on the side with the leak. You can also place a light on the front of the chest (transillumination), which may indicate air has leaked out of the lung and accumulated in the chest.

6. What kind of future complications can we anticipate as a result of this illness?

The majority of babies will have no long-term effects from the air leak itself. The rupture or hole will heal by itself. Any future complications are most likely to occur if the baby is premature or there was another lung problem that required treatment.

7. Are the lungs left weakened from this condition and, if so, in what way?

No, the lungs will heal the tear and recover in almost all cases. If there were other lung problems that were also present, some breathing abnormalities could persist until the lungs are healed from those conditions.

8. After discharge from the hospital, what kind of follow-up will be needed?

As the rupture or tear in the lung is healed at the time of discharge, just routine follow-up with the pediatrician is necessary.

CLAIR SCHWENDEMAN, MD
Neonatology

MECONIUM ASPIRATION

Definition: When the newborn or fetus inhales
meconium (first stool) into the lower
respiratory tract.

1. What caused this condition?

The baby had a bowel movement while still inside the mother's
uterus. Meconium is the name for the first stools that a baby passes.
The meconium gets into the fluid surrounding the baby and can be
swallowed into the lungs or breathing passageways prior to or at the
time of birth. Babies that are under stress or go beyond their expected
due date have a higher incidence of passing meconium while still in
the uterus. Generally, meconium aspiration is seen in babies that are
not premature.

2. Is this condition dangerous, and what kind of damage can it cause?

If the meconium gets into the airways leading to the lungs, it causes a
blockage of the passageways. This stops or impedes the flow of air into

and out of portions of the lungs. This can lead to low oxygen levels or a buildup of carbon dioxide.

If significant, this disruption in the functioning of the lungs can lead to a continued high blood pressure in the blood vessels leading to the lungs. When this occurs, there is further inability of the lungs to get oxygen into the bloodstream and to remove carbon dioxide due to blood bypassing the lungs.

Another common complication of meconium aspiration is the development of a hole in the lung(s). This is called a pneumothorax. Air escapes from the lung into the chest cavity and is trapped between the chest wall and lung. As the air builds up, it compresses the lung and again disrupts normal lung function.

3. What tests are needed to further define the condition?

The presence of meconium is noted when the water is broken either naturally or by the obstetrician. The fluid will have a greenish discoloration. The thickness and degree of discoloration indicates the amount of meconium present. After the baby is born chest X rays will confirm the findings of meconium aspiration if present. A sample of blood called a blood gas along with oxygen-level monitoring (pulse oximeter) will show low oxygen levels and disturbances in lung functioning.

4. What is the treatment?

Prevention is the main treatment. If meconium stained fluid is noted, the obstetrician may infuse sterile salt water into the uterus to dilute the meconium. At the time of delivery, the obstetrician will attempt to clean out the nose and mouth prior to the delivery of the rest of the baby. The baby may then have a breathing tube passed into the trachea, the main passage to the lungs, and suction applied while it is removed.

If the baby has further or continued problems, then additional oxygen and/or a breathing machine may be needed. If a breathing tube is needed, the instillation of a medication called surfactant may be given through it to help break up the meconium and improve the function of the lungs. If the baby has significant breathing concerns, a ventilator called an oscillator may be used.

If the baby develops a pneumothorax, or hole in the lung(s), a drainage tube may be needed. This drainage tube is called a chest tube, and it is placed between the ribs on the side of the air leak to prevent the lung from collapsing.

5. What side effects can occur from the treatment?

The most common early side effect is a hole in the lung(s) from air being trapped by the meconium or from the degree of ventilator support required to get acceptable oxygen and carbon dioxide levels. It is treated as mentioned above.

The lungs can be injured from being on the ventilator. They may develop an inflammatory reaction to the irritation of the meconium and being on the ventilator and high oxygen concentrations. If this occurs, it may delay coming off of the ventilator and additional oxygen. This inflammatory response can occasionally lead to the baby having feeding problems due to increased work of breathing and needing extra oxygen at the time of discharge.

Infrequently, a baby may have severe meconium aspiration along with severe elevations in the blood pressure in the blood vessels leading to the lungs. This may require treatment with a heart-lung bypass (ECMO).

6. How long will it take for my baby to show improvement?

Most babies get better in seven to ten days. A baby with severe meconium aspiration may require a longer hospital stay, potentially up to a month, to be well enough to be discharged.

7. What complications can develop?

The more frequent complications are the same as the side effects from being treated. Holes in the lung (pneumothoraces) or the failure of the blood pressure to lower in the lungs after birth (pulmonary hypertension) may be present and complicate the meconium aspiration. Occasionally, babies may have some inflammation in their lungs that delays their improvement.

8. Can pneumonia develop?

Pneumonia caused by bacteria is not associated with the meconium aspiration itself. Infection may occur in any patient that has a breathing tube in place and receives ventilatory support for a period of time, especially longer than fourteen days.

9. Will this condition weaken my baby's lungs for the future?

Both the presence of meconium and being on a breathing machine with exposure to high concentrations of oxygen can cause an inflammatory response in the lungs. In some cases this can lead to delayed recovery and some lung abnormalities for the first several months of life. Most babies with mild-to-moderate meconium aspiration will not have any long-lasting lung problems.

10.   After discharge from the hospital, what kind of follow-up will be needed?

In most cases, your child's pediatrician will be all that is necessary. In severe cases of meconium aspiration, the baby may be at more risk for developmental delays and a developmental specialist may be required.

CLAIR SCHWENDEMAN, MD
Neonatology

PNEUMONIA–NEONATAL

Definition: Infection of the lungs in the newborn period.

1. What caused this condition?

In the majority of cases, bacteria has gotten into the lungs causing an infection. This can be the only site of the infection, or pneumonia can be present when there is a generalized infection of the bloodstream also.

The bacteria can get into the baby's lungs from the placenta, during the delivery process, or after birth. Occasionally, the pneumonia may be caused by viruses or other infectious agents such as chlamydia, a sexually transmitted infection.

2. How dangerous is this condition, and what complications can occur?

All infections in newborns can be serious and potentially life threatening. Depending on the severity of the pneumonia, the baby may only have fast breathing with need for additional oxygen or could require support with a breathing machine and high levels of additional oxygen.

3. What is the proposed treatment?

As with all bacterial infections, antibiotics need to be started as soon as any infection might be suspected. The antibiotics will ultimately cure the infection. As pneumonia can cause the lungs to not function normally, the baby may need additional oxygen or support with a breathing tube and breathing machine. The length of antibiotic treatment in the hospital is at least seven days and may be more.

4. What potential side effects can occur from the treatment?

Most antibiotics have little to no side effects. Some antibiotics may require blood levels performed to make certain they are in a range to treat the infection, but not cause side effects. If some type of breathing support is needed, holes in the lungs (pneumothorax), or injury to the lungs can occur.

5. How long will it take for my baby to improve once the treatment has begun?

Generally, the newborn will begin to get better twenty-four to forty-eight hours after the antibiotics have been given.

6. What additional diagnostic tests should my baby have?

A chest X ray, blood count, and blood culture are done on babies with suspected pneumonia. Other blood tests that may be done are a measurement of inflammation, c-reactive protein, and a blood gas, which determines how well the lungs are functioning. If a breathing tube is required, a sample of the secretions from the airways may be sent to determine if bacteria are present or not.

7. After the condition is resolved, will my baby be more prone to respiratory tract infections in the future?

No.

8. Do we need to consult with a neonatologist (newborn specialist) or a pulmonologist (lung specialist)?

If the baby requires additional oxygen or breathing support, a neonatologist is consulted. Some babies that have very mild cases or "suspected" pneumonia may stay in the regular newborn nursery under the pediatrician's care.

9. What kind of follow-up will be needed with you in the future?

For mild to moderate cases of pneumonia, routine follow-up with the pediatrician is all that is necessary. In severe cases, a developmental specialist may also monitor your child's progress.

CLAIR SCHWENDEMAN, MD
Neonatology

RAPID BREATHING
(Respiratory Distress
Syndrome/Transient Tachypnea)

Definition: Rapid breathing in the early days of life due to immaturity of the lungs or decreased absorption of fetal lung fluid.

1. What caused this condition?

Rapid breathing (tachypnea) is a sign of an abnormality in the lungs. Causes for the rapid breathing can be lung fluid that did not clear quickly (transient tachypnea of newborn), inadequate levels of a substance (surfactant) in the lungs that prevents them from collapsing (respiratory distress syndrome), or infection (pneumonia).

2. What is actually taking place in the lungs?

The lungs are stiffer than normal and have a decreased ability to get oxygen into the bloodstream and carbon dioxide out. In some cases, there may be gradual collapsing of the small air sacs that, as it progresses, makes the condition worse.

3. How does it differ from pneumonia?

Pneumonia is caused by an infection. This condition is caused by either too much fluid in the lungs after delivery or decreased amounts of a chemical that stops the air sacs in the lungs from collapsing.

4. What tests are needed to further define this condition?

Chest X rays are the main test, but many of these conditions can appear the same on chest X ray. Often the way the baby acts after several hours will determine whether there is just fluid or if there is collapse occurring. Since infection is always a concern, a blood count and blood culture are also almost always done. A blood gas to determine how well the lungs are functioning is also frequently performed.

5. How dangerous is this condition, and can we expect a complete recovery?

If there is extra fluid only, the condition is mild, and the baby generally starts to get better several hours after treatment. If there are decreased amounts of surfactant present, then the baby will most likely need some type of breathing support. Decreased surfactant is a more significant condition with potentially more complications and a longer need for treatment. In both conditions the affected newborn generally makes a complete recovery.

6. What kind of treatment will be needed, and are there any potential negative side effects from the treatment?

In most cases either additional oxygen support and/or breathing support with a machine will be needed. An artificial form of the chemical to prevent lung collapse, surfactant, will be given to babies meeting levels of support to warrant its use. If artificial surfactant replacement is needed, then a breathing tube will be placed into the baby's airway (trachea), and the chemical will be given directly into the lungs. The breathing tube may then be removed or kept in place and a form of breathing support will be started. This breathing support can either be through prongs that go in the baby's nose or by a breathing machine (ventilator) attached to the breathing tube.

As with any abnormality in the lungs and need for breathing assistance, a hole can develop in the lung(s) that allows air to escape from the lung into the chest cavity (pneumothorax). As this air accumulates, it may compress the lungs and cause further worsening of the breathing condition. Many of these leaks require a drainage tube (chest tube) placed into the chest to remove this trapped air. Occasionally, these leaks can also occur within the lungs (pulmonary interstitial emphysema), under the skin, or around the heart. These may require different drainage tubes or special ventilators to treat.

7. How long will my baby need to stay in the hospital?

Depending on the severity and whether it is excess fluid or low levels of surfactant, the baby may stay in the hospital from three days to several weeks. Infants with excess fluid and mild surfactant shortage respond quickly and will have shorter stays. In all cases, the breathing concerns have to be resolved and the baby feeding by mouth prior to going home.

8. Will the treatment or the disorder weaken the lungs in the future and predispose my baby to future respiratory tract problems?

In most babies that are close to their due date or at their due date there are minimal long-term effects on the lungs. The majority of these babies will have no further respiratory concerns.

9. Will I be able to stay in the hospital until my baby is fully recovered?

The usual hospital stay for a mother is two to four days, depending on the type of delivery. Babies with excess fluid have a better chance of being able to be discharged with the mother. Mothers of infants with surfactant immaturity will most likely be discharged prior to the baby's recovery.

10. Will any treatment be needed at home following discharge, and, if so, who will help me administer it?

It is unusual for babies that are not very premature to require any treatments after discharge. More premature babies may require supplemental oxygen, intermittent breathing treatments, or rarely, additional breathing support. Parents of babies with these needs will be trained prior to discharge and often spend one to two days and nights in the hospital with their baby prior to discharge. Sometimes a home nurse may assist or check in regarding the care of the baby after discharge.

11. Do we need to consult with a neonatologist (newborn specialist) or a pulmonary (lung) specialist?

Most babies with breathing issues that require them to be transferred to the neonatal intensive care unit will be cared for by a neonatologist. Pulmonary specialists are generally consulted near discharge if the baby is going to require breathing support at home.

12.   Is this hospital capable of dealing with this disorder, or does my baby need to be transferred to another hospital that is more capable of dealing with difficult illnesses?

This depends on each hospital's capabilities and pediatrician's comfort level in treating sick newborns. Many smaller hospitals will attempt to take care of babies with excess fluid that just need additional oxygen and are stable or improving. If the baby's condition is getting worse and breathing support is needed, that is generally done at larger hospitals that have special areas called neonatal intensive care units (NICUs) and neonatologists (newborn specialists).

13.   After discharge from the hospital, what kind of follow-up will be needed?

This is dependent on the age of the baby at birth. If the baby was near its expected birth date, then usually care with the pediatrician is needed. The more premature the baby was will increase the potential need for pulmonology and developmental specialty care.

CLAIR SCHWENDEMAN, MD
Neonatology

SEIZURES–NEONATAL

Definition: **Convulsive fits or spasms during the first month of life.**

1. What is a seizure?

A seizure is a clinical event (episode) that is the result of excessive activity of a group of nerve cells (neurons) in the brain. There are many different types of seizures (staring, turning the body to one side, jerking of the arms and legs, etc.). The type of seizure a baby has depends upon the baby's age and the part of the brain that the seizure is coming from. Also, the cause of the seizure may determine the type of seizure a baby has.

2. What causes seizures in babies?

Anything that can cause the brain not to work normally can cause a seizure. Common causes in babies include not getting enough blood and oxygen to the brain, bleeding in the brain, infections of the brain, strokes (when the blood flow to a part of the brain is cut off), metabolic problems (such as low blood sugar or calcium), abnormalities in how the brain is formed, inherited problems, or drug withdrawal (such as if the mother used certain drugs or alcohol during the pregnancy—especially on a regular basis). There are other less common causes as well.

3. How are seizures treated, and how effective is the treatment?

Treatment depends upon the cause of the seizure. For example, if the blood sugar is too low, giving sugar typically solves the problem. Sometimes it is necessary to give medication to stop the seizures. The more commonly used medications include diazepam (Valium), lorazepam (Ativan), phenobarbital, and phenytoin (Dilantin). The effectiveness of these medicines at stopping seizures is mainly dependent upon the cause of the seizures. Similarly, how long the baby will need to stay on the medication(s) is often dependent on the cause of the seizures.

4. Are there any side effects to the medicines used in the treatment?

Like any medication, there is always the possibility of side effects. In general, these medications are quite safe. The most common side effect is sleepiness (sedation). This will usually go away once the baby gets used to the medication (typically in three to seven days).

5. What potential harm can the seizures have, and can they cause brain damage?

Many times, it is the presence of brain damage (such as stroke, infection, bleeding in the brain, trauma, and malformations of the brain) that cause the seizures. In these cases, it is the underlying problem that causes brain damage, not the seizure. In some instances, however, especially if the seizures are very long (greater than fifteen to thirty minutes), or they are very frequent, they may cause brain damage.

6. What tests do we need to do to establish any possible underlying cause?

What testing your baby may need will be determined by the circumstances around your baby's seizures. It is likely that your baby will have some blood and urine tests. If it is found that your baby has low blood sugar and giving your baby some sugar solves the problem, then no other testing may be needed. If the doctor is worried about infection, it is likely that he or she will do a spinal tap. If the blood tests are normal and there is not an obvious cause for the seizure, it is likely that your doctor will want to look at your baby's brain, either with a CT or MRI head scan. Your doctor may also want to get a brain wave test (electroencephalogram or EEG).

7. Do you think that the seizures will recur, and what are the possibilities that my baby will outgrow them?

Whether or not the seizures will recur is in large part due to the cause of the seizures. Babies that have had lack of blood or oxygen to brain, strokes, trauma, and conditions where the brain did not form normally tend to have seizures that can be hard to stop and often come back later in life. Babies that are normal except for a family history of seizures in early life or that have had low blood sugar or calcium as the cause of their seizures often do very well, and the seizures typically do not come back.

8. Do we need to consult with a neurologist?

This depends on the cause for the seizures. Babies that have low blood sugar or low calcium as the cause for their seizures do not typically need to be seen by a neurologist. When more serious conditions like stroke, trauma, abnormalities in brain formation, or lack of oxygen occur, follow-up with a neurologist is a good idea.

9. Are there any precautions we need to take when we go home, such as connecting my baby to an apnea monitor?

In most cases, unless there are complicating problems (breathing problems, swallowing problems, etc.), there is no need for special monitoring or precautions. Typically, treating your baby as you would any other newborn is all that is needed.

10.   When do you wish to see my child again regarding this condition following discharge?

When your baby needs to return for follow-up will be dependent on the cause of your baby's seizures. Normally, we will see your baby two weeks after discharge from the hospital. If you see a neurologist in the hospital, he or she will arrange for follow-up if needed. Many times, if follow-up is required, he or she will ask to see your baby one to three months after discharge, but again, this will be determined in large part by the cause of your baby's seizures.

ROY D. ELTERMAN, MD
Neurology

UNDESCENDED TESTICLE(S)

Definition: When one or both testicles do not descend completely into the scrotum.

1. What caused this condition?

There are many theories as to what causes an undescended testis. Some include decreased intraabdominal pressure during the third trimester of pregnancy to push the testis from the abdominal cavity to the scrotum. Some feel that there may be a decreased amount of male hormone such as testosterone during the descent of the testis. However, there is no unifying theory or answer to the cause of undescended testes.

2. Is there a danger of sterility or any other problem as a result of this condition?

If the testicle is undescended only on one side, the fertility rate is the same as a normal population. If there is an undescended testis on both sides, the most current data suggests that fertility is only approximately 65 percent to 70 percent. Testis cancer risk is elevated in *adult* men who have a history of an undescended testis.

3. Will an operation be necessary to correct this condition and, if so, when?

If the testicle is not in the scrotum by approximately nine months of age, then an operation is necessary to position the testicle in the scrotum where it will grow and develop normally. If the testicle is nonpalpable (cannot be felt on examination of the body), then the operation is usually performed at approximately six months of age.

4. When do we need to consult a surgeon?

Generally if a child has an undescended testis, we would like to see the child at a time convenient for the family. Any time between two and six months of age is a good time to have a surgeon initially evaluate the situation.

5. Are there any medicines that can be used to help bring down the testicle(s)?

No.

6. Are there any danger signs that I should look for?

Yes. Most boys who have an undescended testis have a small hernia that coexists with the undescended testis. If there appears to be swelling or tenderness in the groin area suggestive of a bulge or hernia, then this would suggest that the surgery should be done immediately, as this type of hernia can potentially damage or cause loss of the testicle. Rarely an undescended testis can twist (testis torsion) and cause swelling and pain.

7. Following discharge from the hospital, when do you wish to see my baby again?

After discharge, we would like to re-examine the baby in two to three months.

DAVID EWALT, MD
Urology

Part II
Common Conditions in Children and Adolescents

ACNE

Definition: A chronic inflammatory disease of the sebaceous (oil) glands characterized by pimples and pustules occurring primarily on the face, back, and chest.

Author's Comment: There is no need for a teenager to grow up with severe scarring due to acne. Today there are good treatments that can minimize the long-term cosmetic ill effects caused by this condition.

1. What causes this condition to occur in my child?

Acne is triggered by hormone changes in adolescence. Children with acne have oil (sebaceous) glands that tend to produce more sebum (oil). They also have pores that tend to plug more easily. These plugs are made of sebum and dead skin cells. When the pore becomes plugged, bacteria are trapped in the pore, and the pore becomes inflamed, resulting in a pimple. Genetics also plays a role, and some families are more prone to develop acne than others. Unlike what many people think, acne is not due to dirt or not washing your face enough.

2. Is there any way to predict how bad it will get?

Signs that a child may develop more severe acne include earlier age of onset, family history, and being male. As a general rule, males tend to have more severe acne than females. The earlier acne starts (i.e., before age thirteen), the more severe it may be. Children prone to develop bad acne often have family members who had severe or scarring acne. The presence of deeper, tender, cyst-type acne lesions or scarring is a sign of more severe acne, and children with these signs should seek treatment early.

3. What can I do to prevent it from getting worse?

Face washing is not enough. The best thing you can do is to start treatment early. In general, it takes eight weeks for any acne treatment to start working, so if you do not see any improvement from your child's over-the-counter acne treatment after eight weeks, you may need to consider prescription treatment.

Your child should avoid squeezing pimples; this makes the pore more inflamed and increases the risk of scarring. Children should also not scrub their faces harshly or use abrasive cleansers, since this can inflame the skin more. Things that touch or fit tightly against the skin can plug pores, so your child should keep his or her hair, hands, headbands, caps, hair products (gels, hair sprays, etc.), and sports gear off of the face, forehead, shoulders, and back as much as possible.

Products (moisturizers, sunscreens, cosmetics) used on the face and body should be oil free and noncomedogenic (proven not to cause acne). If possible, teens should avoid jobs in places such as fast food restaurants or auto shops, where the skin will be in contact with oil or grease that can aggravate acne.

4. Does diet affect acne?

This is an area of much debate. In general, there are no specific foods that are proven to worsen acne. It is always a good idea to limit junk food as much as possible, but this may not have any bearing on your child's acne. If there is one particular food that consistently seems to worsen your child's acne, then avoiding that food may help.

5. What skin cleanser should be used?

A mild, nonabrasive, nondrying cleanser applied with clean hands or a clean washcloth and warm (not hot) water once or twice daily is recommended. For acne, medicated cleansers containing either benzoyl peroxide or salicylic acid can be used, but they may cause skin irritation or dryness, especially if used in combination with prescription acne medications. Astringents are usually not needed, but may be helpful for teenagers with very oily skin.

6. What about Retin A, benzoyl peroxide, and topical antibiotics?

Retinoids (Tretinoin [Retin A, Renova, or Avita], adapalene [Differin], and tazarotene [Tazorac]) are vitamin A–derived medications and are some of the most effective acne medications that we have. They come in cream or gel forms. Retinoids gently exfoliate the dead skin cells and prevent the first step of acne formation, which is the plugging of the pores. By keeping the pores open, pimple formation is prevented.

Retinoids are effective for all types of acne lesions. Like most acne medications, they are best used on a consistent basis on the entire acne-prone area (rather than spot-treating individual pimples only). Using the medication on all acne-prone areas helps to prevent future pimples from forming. Retinoids work well alone or in combination with other therapies but should be applied sparingly and no more than once daily to limit dryness and irritation, which are common side effects. Because they can make the skin more sensitive to the sun, sunscreens and sun protection should be used. They should not be used by teens who are pregnant.

Benzoyl peroxide is another standard acne therapy. Like the retinoids, it is effective for all types of acne lesions and may be used alone or in combination with other therapies. It has antibacterial as well as antiplugging effects. Benzoyl peroxide is available as a wash or as a leave-on topical (a cream or gel applied to the skin). Dryness is a common side effect and can usually be prevented by applying a gentle moisturizer and stopping the medication for a few days. Some individuals may develop a skin allergy to this medication, so if severe redness or irritation develop, you should consult your child's doctor. Benzoyl peroxide may bleach clothing, towels, or bedding.

Topical antibiotics decrease the acne-causing bacteria (*Propionibacterium acnes*) on the skin but have no effect on plugging of the pores. They work best for inflammatory acne (red bumps, pus bumps, and cysts). It is best not to use topical antibiotics alone as a single therapy. Using topical antibiotics in combination with a retinoid or benzoyl peroxide improves the effectiveness of the medications and makes it less likely that the acne bacteria will develop resistance to the antibiotic over time.

7. What about oral antibiotics?

For teenagers with severe inflammatory acne that does not respond to topical therapy alone, oral antibiotics can be very helpful. As with topical antibiotics, oral antibiotics do not prevent plugging of the pores, so they are not helpful for noninflamed acne lesions, such as black-heads, and are best used in combination with a retinoid or benzoyl peroxide. They should not be used alone as the only acne therapy.

The most commonly used oral antibiotic is the tetracycline family (tetracycline, doxycycline, or minocycline). In general, oral antibiotics are used for a period of several months until the acne is improved and can be controlled with topical medications alone, but use for longer periods of time may be required for some individuals. Courses of less than one month are generally not effective.

These medications are usually well tolerated but can cause nausea if taken on an empty stomach. They can also cause sun sensitivity, so sun protection and sunscreen use is important when taking these medications. For females, taking any oral antibiotic can increase the likelihood of developing a vaginal yeast infection; signs of this include vaginal itching or irritation and a whitish discharge. Oral tetracyclines should not be taken if your child is pregnant. It is common for teenagers to prefer the convenience of oral antibiotics, so they may be tempted to stop their topical medications. For best results, it is very important that they continue using their other medications as prescribed.

8. What about Accutane (oral isotretinoin)?

Oral isotretinoin (Accutane) is the most potent medication currently available for acne. Because this medication can cause birth defects if taken by a pregnant female and because laboratory monitoring is required, this medication should be reserved for severe acne only. It is most effective for severe cystic or scarring acne that has failed to respond to at least three months of maximal combination therapy (oral antibiotic plus a topical retinoid and another topical medication). All patients must be entered into a registry by a physician registered to use this medication, and females must use two methods of birth control to prevent pregnancy. It is not effective for females with hormonal types of acne, such as acne related to polycystic ovary syndrome.

9. When should we consider a dermatologist?

If your child's acne has not responded to over-the-counter therapy or to the medications prescribed by his or her primary care physician, consultation with a dermatologist would be recommended. If your child has severe or scarring acne, if severe acne runs in your family, or if your child develops significant acne at a very young age, you may want to consider seeing a dermatologist sooner.

10. When do you want to see my child again regarding this condition?

Because most acne therapies require a minimum of eight weeks to start working, follow-up two to three months after starting therapy is generally recommended. Earlier follow-up may be needed if problems, such as irritation or other medication side effects, develop. A temporary worsening of the acne four to six weeks after starting treatment is not uncommon and is considered normal; medications should be continued, and the acne typically gets better over the next several weeks.

K. ROBIN CARDER, MD
Dermatology

ANEMIA

Definition: A condition of reduced red blood cells in the circulatory system.

Author's Comment: This is always a worrisome condition in childhood. Anemia can make children sluggish and decrease their capacity to perform. There is no reason why the cause of anemia cannot be fully established and appropriate treatment rendered if necessary.

1. What causes this condition to occur in my child?

Anemia occurs when there are not enough red blood cells to meet the needs of the child. Red blood cells carry oxygen to the various parts of the body. There are three reasons why a child may become anemic.

The first cause is bleeding. If the child is losing red blood cells from the body, whether it is from chronic nosebleeds or from bleeding in the gastrointestinal tract, eventually the red blood cell count will go down, and the child could become anemic.

The second reason why a child may become anemic is if the body is unable to produce sufficient amounts of red blood cells. The most common reason in childhood is a lack of sufficient iron in the diet. This occurs most frequently in children between the ages of one and two who have had a diet made up primarily of cow's whole milk. If the child is not getting sufficient iron in the diet, then the child is not able to make sufficient red blood cells. This can result in severe anemia.

The third reason why a child may become anemic would be if the red blood cells that the child produced do not survive in the body for a normal period of time. Normally, once red blood cells are made, the red blood cells will last in the body for approximately three months. There are a number of conditions that could cause the red blood cells to break down earlier than normal. In general, these are called hemolytic anemias. There are many different types of hemolytic anemia. Some types are inherited and are not correctable. Some types occur after certain viral illnesses and will eventually get better.

2. What tests are needed to better define the condition?

The first step is to measure the amount of hemoglobin and red cells in the body. Then, the physician or the laboratory technician will look at the red blood cells under the microscope. This will often give the physician a clue as to what is causing the anemia.

The physician then might order a number of different tests to determine the diagnosis. For instance, if the physician feels that the child may be losing blood, the physician may order special tests on the stool to look for any signs of blood. The physician also might want to measure the amount of iron in your child's body. There are many tests that can better define the reasons for anemia.

3. How is it treated, and is it correctable?

The treatment for anemia depends on its cause. If the anemia is due to bleeding, then the cause for the bleeding must be determined, and corrective action will be taken. If the anemia is due to an insufficient amount of iron in the diet, then the patient will be placed on supplemental iron, and often a change in diet is warranted. Some types of anemia are not correctable, though the most common forms of anemia are easily correctable.

4. Are there any potential side effects of the treatment?

There is always the possibility of side effects with any treatment, but in general, the treatment of anemia is well tolerated. Certain oral iron preparations may cause some temporary discoloration of the teeth or some belly pains or some constipation. Often, the physician can change the type of iron supplementation to meet your child's needs.

5. What symptoms will my child have as a result of the condition?

In general, the symptoms of anemia are not seen in childhood until the anemia is fairly severe. The signs of anemia generally include fatigue and lack of energy.

6. Do we need to consult a hematologist (blood disorder specialist)?

Most pediatricians are able to diagnose and treat the more common causes of anemia in childhood. Sometimes the pediatrician will request a consultation from a pediatric hematologist for advice in treating anemia.

7. How often will my child need to be tested in the future to see if the condition is improving?

This depends on the cause of the anemia. If the anemia is due to iron deficiency, then the child will be tested several times in the first year or two to make sure that the condition is improving. In other cases of anemia, the scheduling for repeat testing will depend on the cause of the anemia.

8. When do you wish to see my child again regarding this disorder?

The frequency of visits to the doctor for the treatment of anemia will depend upon the cause of the anemia. In general, several trips to the doctor will be required in the first six months to a year if the anemia is due to iron deficiency.

CARL LENARSKY, MD
Hematology

APPENDICITIS

Definition: **Inflammation of the appendix in the large intestine.**

Author's Comment: Whenever a child complains of severe abdominal pains, it is likely that the parent is concerned that the child may have appendicitis. If abdominal pain develops suddenly and the child continues to complain, the doctor should be contacted. It is important that the diagnosis of this condition be established early to avoid having the appendix rupture, which causes more serious problems for the child.

1. How did this condition develop in my child?

The appendix is a leftover of development where the small and large bowel are joined in the right lower quadrant of the child's abdomen. It is hollow, and it opens into the large bowel. The opening is small and susceptible to being clogged by a stool ball (called a fecalith), or it can swell shut when the child has a viral illness somewhere else in the body. The opening of the appendix is surrounded with the same lymphoid tissue that swells in your child's neck when he or she gets a viral illness. The appendix normally has bacteria in its hollow center that are evacuated with the stool. If the opening is blocked, however, the bacteria continue to grow but cannot escape. Pressure builds up, and the bacteria can invade the wall of the appendix, weakening it. If left untreated, the appendix can "rupture," spilling the infection into the wider abdomen.

2. Are there further tests to be done to more fully establish the diagnosis?

The most common test is a CT scan of the abdomen and pelvis. Sometimes a sonogram can also identify appendicitis. There is no single test (or combination of tests) that is 100 percent accurate, so the decision to perform an appendectomy is based on a combination of blood and urine tests, radiology images like a CT scan, and examination by an experienced surgeon. Sometimes, if the diagnosis is in doubt, your child may be admitted to the hospital for a period of observation and/or repeat testing.

3. What is the treatment for this condition?

The definitive treatment is to remove the appendix with an operation. This may be done through an incision in the right lower quadrant of the abdomen or with a laparoscope (which uses three small incisions, one of which is in the belly button). If the appendix has already ruptured and a pus pocket (abscess) has formed around it, the best treatment may be to drain the pus and treat the child with antibiotics first and remove the appendix later (sometimes six weeks later). Many children require intravenous fluids and antibiotics for several hours prior to the operation so they tolerate the anesthesia better.

4. What complications can occur as a result of this condition if left untreated?

The complication that everyone worries about is rupture. If a child has a nonruptured appendix removed, he or she can usually be discharged home without antibiotics in one to two days after the operation. If the appendix has ruptured, however, the child will need five to seven days of intravenous antibiotics after the operation and additional oral antibiotics at home. Even then, children are at much higher risk for abscess formation (usually forms about a week after the appendectomy), which may require drainage with another procedure.

5. What, where, and by whom should the surgery to correct this condition be performed?

The appendectomy is usually performed by a pediatric surgeon in smaller children and by a pediatric or adult general surgeon in teenagers. It must be done in a full service hospital, not a day surgery center.

6. If surgery is necessary, what are the potential complications that can occur?

Local infections in the skin incisions can occur. This appears as bright redness extending more than one-half inch from the edges of the incision or pus draining from the incision. Local infection is treated by removing the outer layer of stitches to allow the area to drain and by antibiotics.

An abscess (a pus pocket formed deep in the abdomen) can occur about a week after an appendectomy for ruptured appendicitis. Formation of an abscess is rare after an appendectomy for nonruptured appendicitis. The abscess is almost always discovered prior to the child going home. If the child still has fever, severe pain, and/or persistently abnormal blood tests greater than one week after the operation, a repeat CT scan of the abdomen and pelvis may be done to check for an abscess. If one is found, one of three treatments will likely be recommended: continued IV antibiotics (for smaller abscesses), drainage by the radiologist using a CT scan for guidance (with the child asleep, a small catheter is inserted into the abscess and left in place until it resolves), or (rarely) another operation for drainage of abscesses that cannot be reached safely by the radiologist.

7. When do you wish to see my child again regarding this condition?

If the appendix did not rupture, one visit to the surgeon two to three weeks after discharge home is sufficient. Most children will be allowed to return to sports or physical education classes after this visit. If the appendix ruptured, an additional visit may be necessary after all antibiotics have been completed.

JOHN L. LaNOUE, MD
Surgery

ASTHMA

Definition: A disorder, usually allergic in nature,
               characterized by spasms and inflammation
               (swelling and irritation) of the bronchial
               tubes (airways) with resultant cough and
               wheezing.

Author's Comment: Fortunately, there are many new treatments out today to treat and prevent asthma flare-ups. With proper medical supervision, children's lives and physical activities do not have to be handicapped by this condition nearly as much as they were in the past.

1. What is the cause of this disorder, and how did my child develop it?

Asthma occurs when a child with certain genes is exposed to an allergic substance in the right amount (unknown) at the right dose (unknown) at the right age (unknown) to produce an allergic reaction in the lung. For most children, asthma is caused by allergy to dust mites, mold, pets, or pollens. Inhaling these allergic substances triggers an allergic reaction that causes airway inflammation.

2. Is it hereditary?

Asthma, together with the other major allergic disorders, eczema and nasal allergy, runs in families in a way that is not completely understood. If one parent or sibling has one of these three disorders, the risk to the child is about 50 percent. If both parents have asthma, allergy, or eczema, the risk is about 80 percent. These problems do not, however, breed true. That is, a child may inherit only one or all three of these allergic diseases.

3. What is the natural course of the disease?

Asthma is extremely variable. Infants, under age two, who have symptoms only with infection, have about a 75 percent likelihood of "outgrowing" the problems. Children who have symptoms triggered by weather changes, exposure to allergic materials, or activity are more likely to have asthma throughout childhood. The older the child is when the asthma first becomes obvious, the less likely it is to be "outgrown." Because the symptoms caused by asthmatic inflammation of the airways are related to the size of the airway, many children seem to "outgrow" their asthma as they approach puberty. For many of these children, asthma returns in their twenties or thirties. Children whose asthma seems to have gone away should be monitored into adulthood.

4. How does infection play a role?

For children of all ages, but especially for young children, viral infection is a major trigger of asthma symptoms and significant asthma flare-ups. Many families have learned to start extra asthma medications at the start of a cold. Sinus infections are also important asthma triggers. Children with asthma who get sinus infections often require additional asthma medications to control symptoms.

5. How is asthma treated, and what are the potential complications of the treatment?

Modern asthma medications are very effective for almost all children. Children with mild, infrequent symptoms have "intermittent asthma" and may be treated with medications to relieve the symptoms of cough, wheezing, or shortness of breath. Because these symptoms are caused by airway spasm, the treatment is to give inhaled "bronchodilators," medications that relax the airway spasm.

Children whose asthma symptoms are more frequent or severe have continued inflammation that triggers the airway spasm. These children with "persistent asthma" require anti-inflammatory medication. The best medications for children with persistent asthma are inhaled corticosteroids or "steroids." It is important to note that these drugs are very different from the "steroids" abused by athletes. When used according to the national and international recommendations, steroids have been proved safe and effective for children as young as six months of age.

Bronchodilators frequently cause hyperactivity or jitteriness. This problem is related to the dose. Because the effectiveness is also related to the dose, children who require frequent treatment during an asthma flare-up experience this side effect. In standard recommended doses, inhaled steroids rarely, if ever, cause side effects.

6. Are there long-term problems that can occur as a result of this disorder?

Inadequately treated asthma causes cough, wheezing, shortness of breath, sick doctor visits, emergency room visits, and hospitalizations. Children with persistent asthma that is not appropriately treated are at risk for lung scarring and progressive loss of lung function.

7. What tests are needed to substantiate the disorder and to determine the severity of an episode?

There is no definitive test for asthma in young children. Lung function testing (pulmonary function tests) is often helpful in older children. A new test, exhaled nitric oxide analysis, measures the waste products of asthmatic inflammation. A very practical and useful test is the response to asthma medications. Cough due to something other than asthma will not improve with asthma medications.

8. How are asthma flare-ups prevented?

Parents need to understand asthma, asthma medications, and what their child's triggers are. Preventing flare-ups starts with avoiding known triggers if possible (e.g., pets that the child is allergic to). When triggers are unavoidable (e.g., pollen or weather changes), parents should be alert to the development of problems and begin a predetermined plan of extra medications to prevent a severe flare-up.

9. Is it necessary to purchase a breathing machine for home use?

Asthma causes very different problems in different children. Some children never experience a severe flare-up of asthma. Others have frequent problems. Inhaled treatments delivered by nebulizer (breathing machine) provide a much higher medication level than metered dose inhalers. Children who experience severe flare-ups benefit from nebulized asthma medications.

10. What symptoms or signs do I need to look for that would indicate my child is getting worse during an episode?

Some signs of severe respiratory problems depend on the age of the child. Infants breathe faster as they worsen. They may also show evidence of working extra hard to breathe by sucking in the muscles between their ribs or above the collarbone. Children of any age who cough with their asthma will have more frequent coughs as they worsen. Shortness of breath, particularly the inability to say a sentence without stopping for breath, is an ominous sign in an older child. During a severe episode, failure to respond to medication is a reason to speak with your doctor or visit the hospital emergency room.

11. Do we need to see an asthma specialist?

Children with mild, intermittent asthma often do well under the care of a pediatrician or other primary care physician. The current guidelines from the U.S. Public Health Service recommend a consultation with an asthma specialist for any child with moderate or severe persistent asthma and for all children under age three with mild persistent asthma.

Any life-threatening asthma episode or hospitalization is justification for specialty care. Several studies have shown that asthma specialists achieve better outcomes and lower costs than primary care physicians in the care of asthma. Because asthma, particularly in children, is usually an allergic disease and most children with asthma have nasal allergy and/or eczema, an allergist is usually the ideal asthma specialist. Pediatric pulmonologists (lung specialists) also treat children with asthma.

12. What kind of follow-up is needed for this condition?

Children with asthma always have the possibility of having asthma symptoms even if they have not had problems for months or years. Some children with asthma hide their symptoms or become so accustomed to having some breathing limitation that they do not notice it. Because undertreated asthma can lead to long-term scarring that cannot be reversed, periodic follow-up is needed even when there are no recognized symptoms.

The frequency of follow-up should be determined by the frequency and severity of symptoms and the amount of medication needed to prevent or treat symptoms. Infants and toddlers who have more than three or four episodes in a year should be seen by their doctor every three months. Young children who take preventive medication every day should see their asthma doctor every three to six months until the teenage years when one or two visits a year is usually sufficient. Older children who do not take daily medications and have episodes that are easily controlled and occur less than once a month should be checked twice a year.

Lung function tests or pulmonary function tests (PFTs) are an important part of asthma monitoring and are strongly recommended by national and international guidelines. Some four- to five-year-olds and most six-year-olds are developmentally able to perform this test. PFTs are very helpful when asthma is difficult to control. PFTs are particularly important after daily medication is stopped to be sure that the child is not having "silent asthma" that is worsening without recognized symptoms.

RICHARD L. WASSERMAN, MD
Allergy and Immunology

ATHLETE'S FOOT
(Tinea Pedis)

Definition: Fungal infection of the foot.

Author's Comment: No need to have your little athlete's feet itching and burning all the time. With proper medical management, this condition can be effectively treated and controlled.

1. What is the cause of this condition, and how did my child develop it?

Athlete's foot is a common fungal infection affecting the soles of the feet. It is more common in teenagers and adults, but can be seen at younger ages in families that are prone to it. The fungus grows best in warm, moist environments like shoes, showers, bathroom floors, gyms, and locker rooms. Walking barefoot (especially in the gym or shower), wearing shoes without socks, or sharing shoes can lead to infection. There is also a family tendency to develop fungal infections, so individuals from affected or susceptible families may be more likely to develop athlete's foot than others.

2. Is it contagious?

Yes. If your child walks barefoot on the same floors as others who have athlete's foot or if he or she shares footwear with affected people, those people can pick up the infection.

3. What medicines are used to treat this condition, and how long are they to be taken?

There are a number of antifungal creams (both over-the-counter and prescription) that are very effective in treating athlete's foot when used twice a day for two to four weeks. For more stubborn cases, oral antifungal pills or liquid taken for one to two weeks can be effective. The feet should be kept dry and should be allowed to air out as much as possible, so open well-ventilated shoes, such as sandals, would be preferred over closed shoes, like boots or athletic shoes.

4. What are the potential side effects of these medicines?

The creams are usually well tolerated but may be irritating if applied to open or cracked skin. Oral antifungal medications can interact with other medications and may affect the liver, so these medications should be monitored by a physician familiar with their use and should be avoided in people with significant liver disease.

5. When would you expect for the symptoms to subside or for the condition to be cured?

Improvement usually takes place within one to two weeks after starting therapy, but two to four weeks may be required for the infection to be completely cleared. A permanent "cure" is difficult, since reinfection is common, unless certain preventative measures are taken.

6. How do we prevent it from spreading to other people, and what can we do to prevent it from coming back?

Because fungus is present on most floors and because certain people are prone to get athlete's foot, reinfection is common. For this reason, preventative therapy is very important both to prevent reinfection and to prevent the infection from spreading to others. The most important thing is to never go barefoot. Plastic shower shoes should be worn in the shower and when walking on bathroom or locker room floors. Keeping feet dry and bringing an extra pair of dry socks to put on after physical education class or sports is also helpful. A topical antifungal cream or spray applied to the feet and between the toes two to three times weekly is also helpful in maintaining improvement and preventing reinfection. If other family members also have athlete's foot, they should be treated as well.

7. What reasons would warrant my calling you back regarding this condition?

If no improvement is seen after one to two weeks of therapy or if drainage, open skin, significant odor, or skin tenderness is noted (especially between the toes), then reevaluation or a change in therapy may be needed.

8. When do you wish to see my child again for this condition?

If your child's feet clear up completely with treatment, no follow-up may be needed, but preventative therapy (see question #6) should be continued.

K. ROBIN CARDER, MD
Dermatology

ATTENTION DEFICIT HYPERACTIVITY DISORDER (ADHD)

Definition: A disorder characterized by an inability to stay focused and attentive.

Author's Comment: This condition, alarmingly, is being diagnosed in epidemic proportions in children. Be sure there is firm evidence for the diagnosis before you embark on a treatment plan. It is important that you keep in close communication with your child's teacher and doctor to maximize the effectiveness of the overall treatment.

1. What causes this disorder?
ADHD is a biological disorder, but the cause is not entirely clear. Parts of the brain that affect attention and activity level may be underactive, and the brain chemicals may be increased or decreased. Other causes of attention differences include head injuries, medications that slow thinking, and sometimes lead poisoning.

2. Is ADHD hereditary or environmental?
ADHD tends to run in some families. If a child has ADHD, other first-degree relatives are five times more likely to also have ADHD.

Sometimes ADHD is recognized in a parent after his or her child is diagnosed. Prenatal exposure to nicotine and alcohol has been associated with increased risk of ADHD. Lead exposure may also potentially cause increased inattention and hyperactivity.

3. What medicines are used to treat this condition?

Most children with ADHD respond to stimulant medications (methylphenidate and amphetamine salt preparations, both short-acting and extended release). There are many brand names to choose from, each of which has some unique feature that your physician may deem most appropriate in the treatment of your child. This class of medication is safe and effective when used according to the doctor's instructions and has been well studied. Stimulants help children with ADHD increase attention span, reduce impulsivity and distractibility, and improve self-monitoring skills.

Other classes of medications may be used if stimulants prove ineffective, or if side effects are problematic. Medication, alone or in combination with behavior therapy, is effective in most children with ADHD.

4. What are the potential side effects of the prescribed medicine that I should look for?

Side effects generally occur in the first couple of weeks of treatment and are frequently temporary. The most common side effects are reduced appetite, sleep disturbance, rebound hyperactivity as the medication wears off, headache, stomachache. Less commonly, jitteriness, mood swings, dry mouth, dizziness, and tics have been reported.

Very rarely, stuttering, increased heart rate or blood pressure, or growth delay may be observed. Children with a personal or family history of a heart condition should be carefully evaluated before starting stimulant medication and during the time he or she is receiving this type of medication.

Side effects of the nonstimulant medications are similar to the stimulant class, but usually they are less pronounced. Both classes of medication may interact with other medications and should be used with caution in individuals with liver problems.

5. Should my child take the medicine on weekends?

Children with ADHD are symptomatic seven days a week. Interference with functioning must be evident in at least two settings, by definition of the disorder. Therefore, children may need medication to control their symptoms during both school and home hours. However, not all children with ADHD need to take medication, and not all need to take medication every day. Parents may help their child feel successful at home without medication by changing the environment and altering their parenting styles to fit their child's needs. Many schools provide environmental modifications for children with ADHD so that treatment with medication is not always necessary.

For those children who take medication to help with schoolwork only, medication may be given on school days only. Many, if not most children with ADHD, take medication seven days per week due to the level of their impairment at home and school. For example, teenagers who take medication for school purposes, but drive without medication on the weekends, may be at increased risk for accidents due to impulsivity and poor judgment. Medication schedules are guided by the child's need for help with self-control, safety, and individual circumstances.

6. Is it dangerous to use the medicine for long periods of time?

Long-term studies reveal that children who stay on medication may fare better than those who discontinue its use. Problems with impulsivity, risk-taking behavior, driving ability, social relationships, and substance use are increased in those who are *not* adequately treated. In addition, there are *no* reports of addiction or dependence on these medications in children who take them in the long term. Several studies suggest that children on stimulants are *not* more likely to abuse other drugs.

Proper monitoring of medication effects and side effects is necessary to ensure appropriate dosing and safety of use over time. Blood pressure, weight, and heart rate should be checked regularly. Delays in growth and development have been shown not to be a significant problem over time, with proper dosing and monitoring.

7. Are there alternative treatments besides medicine?

There are many forms of behavior therapy, and all focus on changing the environment to help the child control his or her behavior. Adults in the child's life learn new techniques to work with the child with ADHD. They help him or her understand what behavior is expected and how to control himself or herself. The family can work with a school or private counselor to set goals with measurable outcomes to track progress. Group therapy is sometimes used to work on social skills, and individual counseling can be useful to address emotional issues which may arise.

There are many "alternative" treatments offered for children with ADHD. You may see advertisements for these products on the Internet, in parenting magazines, and elsewhere. These products range from vitamin supplements, to special diets, biofeedback programs, and special glasses. It is important to realize that none of these remedies have been scientifically proven to be safe or effective treatments for ADHD. Anecdotal evidence or patient "testimonies" are not sufficient to prove effectiveness, so buyer beware!

8. What are the chances of my child outgrowing this condition and when?

The characteristics of ADHD evolve as your child grows. Most children with ADHD in the early elementary years will continue to have the disorder as teenagers, and up to one-half of those teenagers will have symptoms into adulthood. As children mature, their ability to control their behavior and cope with their symptoms matures as well.

Many children discontinue medication in adolescence, but many adults begin taking it when the condition interferes with job performance. Your child's natural history will depend on many factors, but in general, early identification, treatment, and support will predict a more favorable long-term outcome.

9. Are there any other aspects of care that can be helpful in making this condition better?

A thorough evaluation of the child, including physical, psychosocial, and environmental factors is essential. Obtaining appropriate treatment, whether medical, behavioral, or a combination, and proper monitoring are the keys to effective management of your child's ADHD. Early identification and treatment of coexisting conditions is essential, as up to half of children with ADHD have learning problems, emotional disorders, or behavorial disturbances.

10. Do I need to take my child to a psychologist or a neurologist?

Many general pediatricians do a very good job of evaluating children for attention differences. You can ask your child's doctor how comfortable he or she is with this type of evaluation. Your own pediatrician knows your child well and is familiar with your family, which helps with the evaluation process.

In addition to a thorough history of the problem and parental reports, information obtained from a child's teachers is necessary to make a diagnosis. Your child's doctor should have rating forms available to distribute to the school. These forms compare your child to others in his or her age group on a variety of behavioral characteristics and are designed to identify typical or atypical results. Parent forms are also completed to evaluate your child's behaviors. Your pediatrician should be able to explain the results, provide educational materials, and recommendations for treatment, including school modifications, parenting techniques, and behavior modification outlines.

If the child is having academic or social difficulty, consultation with a psychologist may be recommended. If there are concerns regarding developmental or neurological issues, referral to a neurologist or developmental pediatrician may be necessary. For more complicated cases, psychiatric consultation may be recommended.

11. How can the school help?

Your child's school can be very effective in providing educational support and behavior intervention. Classroom modifications can be incorporated to help your child be more successful in the classroom. Your child's teacher should work with you and your pediatrician to develop specific strategies.

When learning issues occur along with ADHD, school diagnostics may evaluate educational needs and recommend special services and modifications as necessary. If your child has a coexisting condition such as a learning difference, he or she may receive services such as individual tutoring, special classroom settings, or an aide, provided by the school.

12. When do I report back to you concerning my child's progress?

Periodic reevaluation and modification of treatment recommendations is essential to effective treatment of children with ADHD. If medication is used, frequent follow-up is necessary to optimize the dosing schedule. It is also important to follow up on recommendations made to the school to ensure that they are in place.

13. How often will you need to see my child in the future regarding this condition?

Medication monitoring is done on a regular basis after the dosage is set, with regular height, weight, and cardiovascular exams. Your pediatrician will set the schedule for appointments. It is important to continue regular visits throughout the year to monitor how well the medication is working and to check for possible side effects. Back-to-school checks are also helpful to outline a plan for the upcoming school year.

LISA W. GENECOV, MD
Developmental Pediatrics

AUTISM

Definition: A condition characterized by impaired social interactions and communication, both verbal and nonverbal, often associated with cognitive behavioral disturbance and deficits.

Author's Comment: The incidence of autism is seemingly on the rise. More pediatric practices around the nation are feeling the brunt of this increasing number. Much research is currently underway to better understand the cause of this disorder and to find better treatments.

1. What causes autism, and why is the incidence on the rise?

Autism is a neurodevelopmental disability that has multiple causes and a strong genetic component. There is no definitive laboratory test to confirm the presence or absence of autism. The diagnosis is made based on a neurodevelopmental profile, defined by the presence of a specified collection of symptoms and behaviors.

Diagnostic criteria have changed over the past fifteen years. Milder variants of autism are now recognized, which accounts for the increasing number of recognized cases. Professionals are also better trained to recognize the early signs of autism, and children are being diagnosed at younger ages. Schools added autism to the list of qualifying conditions that receive special education services in 1991, which may account for part of the increase in the number of children with autism in the school system. In addition, most children with developmental disabilities no longer live in institutions; more children with autism live in our communities and are in our public schools than in the past.

The current estimate of the prevalence of the spectrum of autistic disorders in American children is approximately two to six out of a thousand children, or 0.2 percent to 0.6 percent. This number was reported as 0.5 per 1,000 in 1988 (0.05 percent) and 3 to 4 per 1,000 in the late 1990s (0.3 percent to 0.4 percent). The question remains whether the incidence of autism is really on the rise, or if it is simply more apparent now due to changing diagnostic classifications and heightened public awareness.

Approximately 10 percent to 15 percent of children with autism have a known genetic or medical disorder. Tuberous sclerosis, Fragile X syndrome, and certain metabolic disorders are a few examples. In most children, however, the cause is unknown. A number of genes have been identified that are linked to autism, but diagnostic tests are not yet widely available for most of these conditions. Various nonspecific anatomical changes are seen in the brains of some children with autism, but the factors causing these changes to occur are unknown. Environmental factors may affect prenatal brain development, but more research is needed to answer these and other questions regarding known causes of autism.

2. Is there anything I did as a parent that could have contributed to my child's having this condition?

The original doctor who described classical autism in the 1940s postulated that cold and unnurturing parenting caused a child to develop autism. Current research no longer supports that theory, but the specter of parental responsibility seems to persist. The current consensus among researchers is that autism is caused by the interaction of complex neurobiologic factors, involving one or more genes and that parenting styles do not contribute to the development of autism.

Fetal brain development is affected by a variety of conditions, including alcohol, drug, and tobacco exposure. Two medications, when taken during pregnancy, have been linked to autism: thalidomide and valproic acid. Maternal infections during pregnancy, such as rubella, may also cause autism. The developing brain is especially sensitive during the first eight weeks, often before the pregnancy has been diagnosed. It is possible that exposures during that time period may affect brain development to some extent, but no other definitive environmental factors have been identified.

3. Could autism be related to immunizations?

Multiple scientific studies have revealed *no* evidence to support a link between autism and immunizations (such as against measles, mumps, and rubella [MMR]) or thimerosal (a vaccine preservative that contains ethyl mercury). Multiple stories in the media have kept these myths in the public eye, but scientific reports have failed to support the claims. In addition, the use of thimerosal as a vaccine preservative was discontinued several years ago, eliminating this issue as a reason not to vaccinate.

4. Are there any diagnostic tests needed to further define this disorder?

Several types of tests may be performed as part of a comprehensive evaluation. A comprehensive developmental assessment, measuring a child's language, motor, cognitive and adaptive skills should be performed on all children suspected of having autism. Specially designed tests are also used as part of the evaluation.

Further medical diagnostic testing may be indicated based on findings from the history and physical exam. These tests may include blood work for specific genetic and metabolic disorders, electroencephalogram (EEG), or MRI scanning.

5. What is the current treatment, and how effective is it?

The most effective treatment for autism is a comprehensive program including developmental, educational, and behavioral therapies. Early intervention in language, social, and cognitive development is important in maximizing the child's developmental potential. Individual speech/language therapy, developmental therapy, and/or motor therapy may be recommended. Child-centered therapeutic approaches are often more effective. Additional methods, such as sign language, picture exchange systems, and communication devices are often used to augment spoken language.

Involvement in a specialized preschool program is recommended, not only for academic instruction, but also for socialization to the classroom. A specifically designed curriculum for children with autistic disorders focuses on the specific difficulties children have with communication, socialization, behavior, and transitions. Social skills training is often effective in facilitating interactions with others.

Behavioral intervention involves analyzing problem behaviors and developing strategies to help the child adapt and respond to the environment. Applied behavior analysis and relationship-based intervention models focus on eliminating unwanted behavior and teaching appropriate skills in communication, socialization, and learning.

Many families participate in complementary or alternative medical treatments. Anecdotal reports of children who dramatically improved after treatment with certain medications or therapies can be found in books, on the Internet, or from other parents. Often, no scientific evidence exists to support these claims, but due to the nature of the condition and the lack of specific treatments for autism, these therapies often gain popularity and then fade when a new alternative therapy arises. Some examples of these treatments include antifungal medications, high-dose vitamins, secretin, steroids, heavy metal chelation, and gluten- and lactose-free diets. It is important to review any treatments not prescribed by your child's doctor with him or her before beginning, both to receive objective evidence of effectiveness and to explore any unexpected side effects that treatment may cause.

6. Do we need to see a developmental pediatrician and/or a neurologist for this disorder?

Early screening and diagnosis are essential in improving the outcome of children with autism. There are several screening tools available that may be administered in a pediatrician's office. If the screen is positive, referral to a comprehensive evaluation center is important. There are many conditions that can present a similar profile, and determining the presence or absence of autism is sometimes difficult. A multispecialty evaluation is important in making a definitive diagnosis of autism. If a comprehensive center is not available in your area, consultation with an experienced clinician—a developmental pediatrician, a neurologist, or psychiatrist—may be recommended.

7. How do we get my child's school involved?

Children with autism are eligible for special education services through the public schools beginning at the age of three through twenty-one. Contact your school district's special education division to request a full individual evaluation. After testing is completed, you will meet with a school committee to receive the results and their recommendations for services. Parents are considered full partners on the committee. The committee will write an Individual Education Plan that outlines specific services your child will receive and goals for learning. This may include additional services, such as speech therapy, as well as classroom placement. The plan will be reviewed and revised on an annual basis, or on request if your child is not making the expected progress on the plan. A complete reevaluation takes place every three years.

The Individuals with Disabilities Education Act provides that children with disabilities (including autism) are educated in the least restrictive environment. Children with disabilities may be placed in regular classrooms with a few special services. At times, a self-contained special education classroom is the best placement. It is up to the school committee and you, the parents, to agree on the best classroom setting for your child.

If there is a disagreement with the committee's recommendations, parents are urged to delay signing until there is full agreement. If an acceptable plan cannot be agreed upon, a complaint is filed, and a due process hearing is requested.

8. How do we as parents get help and counseling?

A comprehensive evaluation center will provide parent education, support, and resources. Understanding the diagnosis and knowing how you can impact your child's future are critical in developing a family plan of intervention. Social work services may help families find financial support, respite services, and other resources. Connecting with other families who have children with autism can help provide a network of understanding and information. Online communities are also available as a resource, allowing families to connect on a more global basis. Family, marital, or individual counseling may sometimes be recommended.

9. What type of follow-up is needed?

Periodic follow-up is important in assessing your child's developmental progress and evaluating therapeutic interventions. At times, other pediatric specialists may be consulted, such as a neurologist, a geneticist, or a psychologist. As your child grows and enters new phases of development, new challenges may arise. Consultation with your pediatrician can help determine what other professionals should be involved.

LISA W. GENECOV, MD
Developmental Pediatrics

BACK PAIN

Author's Comment: Back pain in children is more common than previously thought. More than 50 percent of children experience some back pain by fifteen years of age. Backaches in childhood can sometimes be more serious than a muscle strain. If the symptom persists, have it thoroughly evaluated by your child's doctor.

1. What are the possible causes for this condition?

The causes are many and varied. Back pain may result from mechanical disorders, such as muscle strain, disk herniation, or vertebral fracture, or developmental disorders, such as spondylolysis (vertebral stress fracture), scoliosis, and kyphosis (postural roundback). Other causes include underlying spinal column abnormalities, infectious or inflammatory conditions, and benign or malignant tumors.

2. What tests can better define the cause of the problem, and is now the right time to perform these tests?

A thorough, detailed history provides the most important information when evaluating children with back pain. The history, along with a careful physical examination, will give your doctor the information needed to order the appropriate testing, if necessary. X rays are typically ordered to rule out structural or developmental causes. Advanced imaging may include CT scan or MRI, if necessary. Infectious or inflammatory conditions may be evaluated with laboratory blood tests. The timing of these tests depends on information gained from the history and physical examination.

3. What can be done to make the condition better?

The treatment of back pain in children depends completely on the cause. Initial treatment for the most common causes of your child's back pain usually includes temporary activity modification and physical therapy to stretch and strengthen the back muscles and to stretch the hamstrings.

4. Are there any medicines that can be used?

Tylenol or anti-inflammatory medicines, such as ibuprofen (Motrin) or naproxen (Aleve), may be used for most mechanical and inflammatory causes of back pain. Antibiotics should be used to treat infections causing back pain. Typically, narcotic pain medicine is not necessary in the treatment of children with back pain.

5. If medicine is used, what are the potential side effects?

In proper doses, these medications have few side effects. Anti-inflammatory medicines should be taken with food to minimize side effects, such as upset stomach. Long-term use of anti-inflammatory medications can lead to stomach ulcers. Certain antibiotics can also cause upset stomach or diarrhea.

6. What kind of exercise limitations should be enforced?

This depends on the cause of back pain. Most musculoskeletal causes can be treated with a brief (one to four weeks) period of rest and stretching, followed by gradual return to activities. Exercises that are persistently painful should be avoided. Stress fractures (spondylolysis) are treated with two to four months of running and jumping restrictions. For more serious causes of back pain, such as fracture, infection, or tumor, your child should avoid all rigorous activity until cleared by your orthopedic surgeon.

7. Do we need to consult with an orthopedist or a chiropractor?

With pain that persists or is disabling, consultation with an orthopedist is important to accurately diagnose the cause of back pain and to order further tests, if necessary. For the most common causes of back pain in children, physical therapy is necessary for low back stretching and strengthening, and hamstring stretching. Some individuals elect to use a chiropractor for the stretching activities. Occasionally, gentle manipulation of the spine may be therapeutic.

8. When do you wish to see my child again for this problem?

Your orthopedic surgeon will need to see you and your child to review test results and to evaluate the response to therapy. Follow-up is typically every six to twelve weeks until your child's symptoms resolve.

RODERICK CAPELO, MD
Orthopedics

BEDWETTING (Enuresis)

Definition: Involuntary wetting of the bed.

Author's Comment: This is frequently an embarrassing condition for children when they reach grade-school age. Once you have your child evaluated by the doctor, there is usually an effective treatment that can be prescribed.

1. What causes this condition to occur in my child?

Nighttime wetting occurs when urine production during the night exceeds the bladder's ability to hold that urine (i.e., the bladder's capacity). There are multiple causes of bedwetting. This problem tends to run in families, with some studies demonstrating an incidence of over 40 percent if one parent experienced nocturnal enuresis and over 70 percent if both parents did. Nocturnal enuresis can also be seen in children with daytime wetting problems, urinary tract infections, diabetes, sleep apnea, or constipation as well as other medical problems.

2. How long will it last?

Enuresis occurs in approximately 10 percent to 20 percent of five-year-olds. We know that there is a 15 percent chance of the problem resolving itself per year. Persistence of this problem into young adulthood is thought to be around 1 percent.

3. Is there any treatment for this condition, and at what age is it necessary?

Treatments for nocturnal enuresis can involve behavioral alterations (better daytime bathroom behavior, alteration of nighttime fluid consumption), treatment of constipation, alarm therapy, or medication (desmopressin, imipramine, or others).

Treatment needs to be individualized as there can be many contributing factors to bedwetting. It is important to keep in mind that each of these therapies addresses a different aspect of nocturnal enuresis. A treatment to reduce nighttime urine production will not likely help a patient with the primary problem of a reduced bladder capacity.

Intervention should be introduced when the enuresis is of concern to the child and may be impacting his or her self-esteem. It is not recommended to start treatment before five years of age. Of course, parental concern is also a reason to begin treatment. Usually treatment is started around seven to eight years of age.

4. How successful is the treatment?

Behavioral therapy by conditioning or bladder training (i.e., alarm therapy) is very effective, with some studies suggesting around a 70 percent success rate. Medical therapy with desmopressin or imipramine can reduce the frequency of enuresis; however, very high rates of relapse have been reported after stopping the treatment.

5. Are there any side effects from the treatment?

In general, these treatments are well tolerated, although there are specific concerns with each of the medicines that should be discussed with the prescribing physician or pharmacist.

6. What further diagnostic tests are needed to better define the problem?

A urinalysis is helpful in the initial evaluation of a child with bedwetting. Information such as the presence of urinary tract infection, inability to concentrate urine (leading to too much urine production), or glucose in the urine can give insight into the source of the problem. Other tests your doctor may wish to order include an ultrasound of the kidneys and bladder, or bladder X rays (voiding cystourethrogram). Specialized testing in a urologist's office can be performed to gain information about your child's urine flow and bladder function. An MRI of the spine may be ordered if there are concerns about certain neurological conditions that may be underlying this condition.

7. Are there possibly psychological factors involved?

Psychological factors are not thought to be among the leading causes of bedwetting. However, the impact of prolonged bedwetting on a child's self-image and social interactions is an important consideration and should weigh on the decision to be evaluated. Children with ADHD have a higher incidence of bedwetting and may be more difficult to treat.

8. Do we need to consult a urologist?

A pediatric urologist can be very helpful in evaluating children with enuresis that have not responded to basic behavioral changes or initial medicinal interventions. Additionally, children with daytime problems (daytime accidents) or urinary tract infections would benefit from urologic consultation. Many pediatric urology offices are equipped with specialized testing equipment that can help evaluate nonresponsive or more complicated children.

9. When do you wish to see my child again regarding this condition?

It is important to allow a reasonable period of time following any intervention to assess success or failure. Typically, six to eight weeks following the initial visit would be a good time to reevaluate your child.

ADAM G. BASEMAN, MD
Urology

BELLYACHES
(Recurrent Abdominal Pain)

Author's Comment: This is one of the most common complaints in childhood. If the symptom persists or is severe to the point of interfering with your child's daily activities, it warrants a complete evaluation by the doctor.

1. What are the possible causes for this condition?

Recurrent abdominal pain is a common complaint in children ages four to fourteen. Although there is no known solitary cause, "functional" abdominal pain is likely a combination of motility (the colon's ability to contract), sensory, dietary, immunological, social, and psychological processes.

Typically, the pain is located around the belly button and seldom localizes to the right, left upper, or lower abdominal regions. Rarely, vomiting, diarrhea, or constipation may accompany the pain, but they are usually mild and temporary. The symptoms may or may not be related to meals, specific foods, activities, stress, or school. The child might miss school or activities on a recurring basis because of the pain.

2. What further tests need to be done to substantiate the diagnosis and to make sure this condition does not need further attention?

A good history and physical exam are adequate in most cases. However, a reasonable evaluation may include blood tests to check for anemia, liver and pancreas irritation, and celiac disease (gluten sensitivity). Stool and urine tests may also be ordered. Your doctor might also consider an ultrasound, CAT scan, or upper GI series (special X ray).

3. Do you think the condition could be one that may require surgery?

Unless the tests show gallstones, kidney stones, kidney obstruction, appendicitis, or an abdominal mass, surgery is not required.

4. Are there any medicines that can make the condition better?

There is no drug that is consistently reliable. However, it is important to acknowledge that the pain is real, minimize secondary loss of function such as school absenteeism or restriction of activities, and address social or environmental stressors that may be contributing to the condition.

5. How long do you think that the abdominal discomfort will last?

Once the diagnosis has been discussed with you, symptoms usually resolve in two to six weeks in 30 percent to 50 percent of patients. Interestingly, 30 percent to 50 percent of these children may have similar symptoms as adults, but rarely do the symptoms alter lifestyle or limit activity. Some of these children may also be more susceptible to headaches, backaches, and other nonspecific ailments as adults.

6. What things do I look for that would suggest the condition is getting worse?

The following symptoms would merit reevaluation:

- Fever
- Weight loss
- Persistent vomiting, diarrhea, or constipation
- Bloody stools or skin tags (bits of hanging skin) about the anus
- Loss of appetite or symptoms brought about by eating
- Joint pain
- Rash
- Awakening from a sound sleep with pain
- Headache or dizziness
- Change in urinary habits
- Emotional instability, anxiety, or depression

7. When should I call you back concerning my child's condition?

Call back if any of the above symptoms develop, or if reasonable attempts to restore the child's routine to a more normal, functional lifestyle fail after a six- to eight-week period. This would include normal school attendance, interaction with family and peers, as well as play and social activities.

8. What kind of follow-up is needed?

If the pain resolves within a short period of time, routine pediatric visits are adequate. If the symptoms persist, more frequent visits might be required. Some tests may have to be repeated after several months of unresolved pain.

KENDALL O. BROWN, MD
Gastroenterology

BLADDER INFECTION
(Cystitis)

Definition: Infection of the bladder.

Author's Comment: Make sure you do all the follow-ups and diagnostic tests that your doctor requests regarding this condition. You do not want this to lead to a chronic condition in your child later on in life.

1. What causes this condition, and how did my child contract it?

Bladder infections are caused by bacteria that grow in the urinary bladder. Almost all bladder infections come from bacteria that enter the bladder through the urethra, which is the urinary channel from the bladder to the tip of the penis in the male and to the vulvar area in the female. Bacteria are able to move, and they travel up the urethra and enter the bladder. The bacteria originate from the colon and/or the child's stool.

2. Now that my child has this condition, what are the chances that it will come back?

Cystitis is very uncommon in males. If the male has a history of cystitis or infection of the bladder, this is a potential sign of a serious underlying abnormal condition of the bladder or male urethra. The likelihood it will recur if the child does have a significant condition is quite high. In females cystitis is much more common because the urethra or urinary channel from the bladder to the surface of the skin is much shorter, and it is much more likely that bacteria can enter the bladder. In addition, there are more bacteria in the vaginal area than there is on the surface of the penis in the male unless the male is uncircumcised. The chances of it recurring in females over two years after having one infection is approximately 20 percent.

3. What is the treatment for this condition, and how long will it be continued?

The treatment for bladder infection includes increased fluids, specific antibiotics to eradicate the bacteria from the bladder, frequent urination to empty the bladder as completely as possible, and meticulous genital hygiene. Generally, the antibiotic treatment is between three and ten days. However, increased fluids, frequent voiding, and meticulous genital hygiene should be continued after the infection has cleared.

4. If medicines are used, what are the potential side effects?

Any antibiotic medication can cause an allergic reaction with a skin rash. In a small number of cases medication can cause abdominal discomfort, diarrhea, and yeast infections in the vaginal area in females. However, each antibiotic has specific side effects, and you should inquire about this with your doctor or pharmacist.

5. How long will the symptoms last once treatment is started?

The most common symptom of bladder infections is burning with urination and urinary frequency. Once specific therapy is begun, the burning with urination and frequent urination usually will resolve in twenty-four to seventy-two hours.

6. Are there any X ray studies that can determine any underlying anatomical reason for this type of infection?

Yes. There are a number of X ray studies that are typically performed to evaluate the kidneys and bladder after a bladder infection. However, there is much controversy as to when and what tests need to be performed. Typically, a renal and bladder ultrasound is performed to evaluate the kidneys and look for kidney stones. A voiding cystourethrogram (VCUG) is typically used to evaluate the bladder. A small catheter is inserted into the bladder, and the bladder is filled with a dye to look for a condition known as vesicoureteral reflux or backwash of urine up to the kidney.

If a boy has a urinary tract infection, even one, most physicians would recommend a renal ultrasound and VCUG. In females, if the child has one infection under the age of five, most urologists at this time would recommend an evaluation with renal ultrasound and VCUG. If the child is over age five, generally the workup will commence after two infections. However, once again there is a great deal of controversy and a significant amount of research being performed in this area to further tailor the needs of these studies.

7. If there is an anatomical abnormality, will we need to see a pediatric urologist?

Yes. If there are any anatomic abnormalities such as vesicoureteral reflux, obstruction of the urinary tract, renal or bladder stones, or any other abnormality of the bladder or kidneys, the patient and family should see a pediatric urologist shortly thereafter.

8. When do I need to bring in follow-up urine specimens to see if the medicines are working?

After the child has been off antibiotic medications for treatment of the urinary tract infection, it is common to perform a follow-up urinary specimen approximately ten days to two weeks after the last dose of antibiotic.

9. When should I call you back regarding this condition?

After the initiation of antibiotic medication there should be a call back in approximately forty-eight hours to confirm that the child is responding to the antibiotic medication and any other treatments prescribed by the physician.

10. When do you wish to see my child again for a follow-up exam?

If treatment of the urinary tract infection has been completed and X ray studies have been performed, follow-up will be determined by the findings on the X ray studies. If the X ray studies are normal, then the child should be followed up only if he or she has symptoms of a urinary tract infection.

If the child has repeated infections with normal X rays, the most common reason for this is urinary or stool holding and incomplete emptying of the bladder. If that occurs, consultation with a pediatric urologist would be recommended.

If there are abnormalities identified on the X ray studies that confirm an anatomic reason for the infection, then follow-up would depend on the condition and recommendations by the pediatric urologist.

ADAM G. BASEMAN, MD
Urology

BLOOD IN URINE
(Hematuria)

Author's Comment: Frequently, this condition is picked up as part of a routine wellness exam. It can be a representation of a serious underlying condition, so be sure to do all the follow-up testing that your doctor requests.

1. What are the possible causes of this condition?

Hematuria can be caused by diseases in the bladder or kidneys. Bladder diseases, such as a urinary tract infection or bladder stones, are accompanied by urgency and pain with urination. Kidney diseases include inflammation of the kidney, infections, structural abnormalities, kidney stones, elevated urine calcium levels, and cysts. Inflammation of the kidney is common and can occur as a result of a recent streptococcal infection of the throat or skin (poststreptococcal glomerulonephritis).

Blood in the urine can appear pink, red, or dark brown in color. It can also be present in such scant amounts so as not to alter the color of the urine.

2. Are any of the causes potentially dangerous for my child?

Poststreptococcal glomerulonephritis is complicated by high blood pressure (hypertension) and may require hospitalization to treat elevated blood pressures.

Another dangerous cause of hematuria is kidney stones. Kidney stones are very painful and will require medical attention to treat the pain and remove the stone. A pediatric urologist will surgically remove the stone, if necessary. After the removal or passage of the kidney stone, your child will need further evaluation to find the cause of the kidney stone and receive treatment. Without treatment, many kidney stones will recur. Kidney infections require oral or intravenous antibiotics. With delayed treatment, kidney infections can lead to kidney scars, reduced kidney function, and later hypertension.

3. Is there any specific treatment for this disorder, and are there any activity restrictions that need to be imposed?

Hematuria, per se, is not harmful to the kidney and does not require any specific treatment. However, certain conditions associated with hematuria may be harmful and require treatment. For example, kidney stones require immediate treatment. Kidney diseases that are accompanied by protein loss in the urine may require specific medications to curb the loss of protein. In general, there are no activity restrictions placed on patients with hematuria. Any patient able and willing to engage in physical activities is allowed to participate within the limits of general safety.

4. What diagnostic tests should be done to better define the cause of this problem?

The diagnostic tests ordered by your physician for your child with hematuria will help pinpoint the source of the blood in the urine. A simple office urine dipstick test and microscopic examination will help determine whether the blood comes from the kidney or bladder. Blood tests will help to determine the nature and severity of the associated kidney disease. A kidney ultrasound test will often be ordered to ascertain the size, shape, and structure of the kidney.

In rare instances, a kidney biopsy may be required to determine the cause of the hematuria. Your pediatrician may refer your child to a pediatric nephrologist (kidney specialist), who will discuss and determine whether a kidney biopsy is necessary.

5. Will my child outgrow this condition?
The duration of hematuria depends upon its exact cause. In most instances of poststreptococcal glomerulonephritis, the hematuria will resolve on its own over time. However, in other instances of more severe inflammatory kidney diseases, the hematuria may not resolve until the inflammatory condition is medically treated. In certain situations, the hematuria may persist chronically. It is important to remember that hematuria, in itself, is usually not harmful to your child or the kidneys.

6. Do we need to see a nephrologist (kidney specialist) or a urologist (urinary tract specialist)?
Hematuria that arises from bladder diseases is best followed by a pediatric urologist, while hematuria that arises from kidney diseases should be followed by a pediatric nephrologist. Most cases of hematuria in children arise from kidney diseases. Therefore, if your child has persistent hematuria, your pediatrician will likely refer your child to a pediatric nephrologist. In contrast, most cases of hematuria in adults arise from bladder diseases and are referred to an adult urologist.

7. What symptoms pertaining to this condition would warrant my calling you back again?

Urine that is visibly bloody is a hallmark of more severe kidney disease and should warrant medical attention. Any type of pain in the flanks (lower back) or pain with urination, particularly when associated with a fever, may indicate a kidney stone or kidney infection and requires immediate medical attention. Also, if your child's hematuria is associated with joint pain; muscle aches; a rash; or facial, abdominal, or leg swelling, systemic inflammatory disease may be associated with the hematuria. In this case, your pediatrician will refer your child to a nephrologist.

8. How often do you want to test the urine for blood in the future, and when do you wish to see my child again regarding this condition?

An office urine dipstick test will be performed during each visit to your child's pediatrician or, if necessary, the pediatric nephrologist. The urine dipstick is a quick yet sensitive method to detect blood in the urine. The frequency of visits will depend upon the nature and severity of the kidney disease.

Mild or benign kidney conditions, such as poststreptococcal glomerulonephritis or elevated urinary calcium, may only require visits every three to six months. However, more severe kidney disease will require medical therapy and more frequent follow-up visits, up to every two to four week visits.

ALBERT QUAN, MD
Nephrology

BLOOD VESSEL BIRTHMARK
(Hemangioma)

Definition: A superficial collection of blood vessels on the skin.

Author's Comment: Take heart! Many of these unsightly birthmarks fade significantly over time. Keep in mind, some get worse before they get better. Rarely, some of these do not regress to a desirable level and require more aggressive therapy at a later date.

1. What causes this condition to occur, and how did my child acquire it?

Hemangiomas are common birthmarks made of the cells that line our blood vessels. They occur at random, but are more common in females, premature babies, and twins. The cause is unknown.

2. Did something happen during the pregnancy that might have caused it?

These birthmarks are not caused by anything a mother ate, did, or did not do during pregnancy.

3. Is it potentially dangerous?

If the hemangioma is large; deeply ulcerated; or involves the eyelids, lips, or nose (such that it affects vision, eating, or breathing), then problems may occur, and treatment should be sought. Larger lesions on the face or over the buttocks and lower spine can be problematic and may be associated with neurological or other problems. Children with more than one hemangioma are at risk to develop internal hemangiomas, which can be serious in some cases.

4. What is the usual course of these birthmarks?

The lesions are usually small or unapparent at birth, then grow rapidly over the first few months of life. At around six to twelve months, the hemangioma stops growing, and the lesions involute (become flatter and less red) slowly over the next several years. As a general rule, 50 percent of lesions have improved by age five years.

5. What kind of treatment is needed, or will it fade on its own?

Small or thin lesions often fade well over time and require no treatment. Larger, ulcerated, or more raised hemangiomas may require treatment with oral steroids to halt the growth of the lesion and limit disfigurement or complications. Oral steroids are very helpful but are not recommended for use in all hemangiomas. Side effects include increased appetite, weight gain, fussiness, disruption of the sleep schedule, high blood pressure, and increased susceptibility to infection.

For deep or stubborn ulcerations, treatment may include ointments, special dressings, pain medication, or laser treatment.

6. Will it eventually leave any disfiguring mark?

Some smaller hemangiomas may resolve without a trace, but most lesions leave behind some discoloration (red or white) or skin texture change. Residual redness can be treated with the pulsed dye laser. Lesions that are more raised can leave residual sagging skin. For this, surgery may be required to remove the excess skin. Deep ulcerations can leave areas of whitish scarring once healed. Larger lesions involving the nose or lip can alter the normal shapes of these structures, resulting in disifigurement.

7. Do we need to consult with a dermatologist regarding this condition?

A dermatologist should be consulted for larger hemangiomas (particularly on the face or tailbone area) and hemangiomas that are painful, bleeding, or have the potential to affect breathing, eating, or vision.

8. What kind of follow-up is needed?

For smaller lesions, no follow-up may be needed unless sagging skin or residual discoloration remains at around three to five years of age. If oral steroid therapy is needed or if ulceration is present, then more frequent follow-up (sometimes as often as once a week) may be needed. Any change that is worrisome to parents merits a phone call to the doctor and possibly follow-up in the office.

K. ROBIN CARDER, MD
Dermatology

BOIL
(Carbuncle)

Definition: A painful nodular area of inflammation in the skin, frequently with a central core of pus.

Author's Comment: Some children are more prone to this condition than others. If your child falls into this category, pay more attention to the child's personal hygiene and talk to your doctor about what else can be done to prevent recurrences.

1. What caused this condition to occur in my child?

Bacteria that are normally present in the environment can cause boils if they gain access to the deeper layers of the skin through a break in the skin, such as a cut or bug bite. It can be thought of as a pimple that, instead of draining to the outside, expands into the underlying tissue.

2. Is it contagious, and, if so, how do I prevent it from spreading to other people?

Contact with the drainage from boils can spread the infection but usually causes problems only if the bacteria get into a break in the skin of another person. If they are occurring in multiple family members, everyone may need to undergo some form of treatment such as ointment in the nasal passages (this is unusual).

3. What is the treatment?

Small boils (less than 1 inch in diameter) that drain on their own may only need antibiotic treatment. Larger ones or those that enlarge or fail to resolve with oral antibiotics may need drainage in an emergency room or operating room as well as intravenous antibiotics. Sometimes a small drain (which looks like a rubber band) is left in for a few days to allow the body to heal the center. The area is then washed twice a day with warm soapy water, and gauze is placed over the area to catch the drainage.

4. If medicines are prescribed, how long should they be used?

Antibiotics are generally given for ten to fourteen days and must be completed per your doctor's instructions, even if it appears to have healed earlier.

5. Are there any complications or side effects that can occur as a result of the treatment?

The antibiotics can sometimes cause diarrhea. This can often be improved by feeding the child yogurt with live cultures (not frozen) to reestablish normal healthy bowel bacteria.

6. How effective is the treatment in eradicating the condition?

The combination of drainage and antibiotics is very effective in resolving the boil, but if they occur three or more times, additional testing may be necessary to check the immune system.

7. What can be done to prevent a recurrence of this disorder?

If boils occur more than once, your doctor may have you put antibiotic ointment in the child's nose and around the anus to decrease bacterial colonization.

8. What kind of follow-up is needed?

If a drain is placed, the surgeon will usually remove it in the office in three to five days.

JOHN L. LaNOUE, MD
Surgery

BREAST ENLARGEMENT IN MALES (Gynecomastia)

Definition: Abnormal breast enlargement in a male.

Author's Comment: This can be an embarrassing condition for children, especially for teenagers. It occurs in approximately 30 percent to 50 percent of teenage males. In most cases, straightforward information and reassurance go a long way in bolstering the child's self-esteem.

1. What causes this condition to occur in my child?

When gynecomastia occurs in a teenage boy, it is almost always part of normal pubertal maturation. Likely, it is due to the newly begun production of testosterone and the temporary conversion of some of this testosterone into estrogen. The estrogen causes the enlargement of the breast tissue.

Obesity can exacerbate the problem, both by accelerating the conversion of testosterone into estrogen (which occurs in the fat cells) and by adding extra padding, making the tissue contour appear bigger.

In very rare instances, gynecomastia can be caused by disorders resulting in excess estrogen production in boys, including liver dysfunction, testicular tumors, or chromosomal abnormalities.

2. Is there something hormonally wrong with my child?

Generally, there is not. In the usual case, the breast tissue does not grow any larger than 2 inches in diameter, persists no longer than 18 months (but usually about 6 months), and occurs in the middle stages of puberty. Boys in whom the signs are outside these parameters should be evaluated for hormonal abnormalities.

3. What can be done to correct this condition?

In the vast majority of cases it is self-limited, meaning it occurs for a period of time, and then typically goes away. It requires no specific therapy except for time. In the rare cases of underlying hormonal abnormality, the underlying problem would need to be identified and treated.

If the gynecomastia persists beyond two years or correction of the underlying illness does not lead to the resolution of the breast tissue, then surgical removal of the tissue is the usual treatment.

4. Are there any tests needed to further define the cause of this disorder?

If the breast tissue persists longer than eighteen months, if it is large, or if it does not occur during puberty, your pediatrician will want to schedule a visit. Lab testing may be needed to diagnose some of the rare causes of gynecomastia.

5. Do you think the breasts will grow any larger?

Generally, the true breast tissue does not get larger than 2 inches in diameter. The tissue may appear larger if there is a significant over-laying layer of fat.

6. How should I counsel my child?

Let your son know that close to half of boys will develop some degree of breast development during the time of puberty. Counsel him to let you know if the tissue is enlarging or not resolving with time. With growth of the breast tissue, there can be some tenderness even to light touch; let your pediatrician know if the tenderness is increasing. Weight management skills should be reiterated. Let him know that he is not "turning into a girl." This is actually a secret fear of many boys when they experience gynecomastia. Let him know that the pediatrician is a good resource for discussion about this should his concerns persist.

7. Do we need to see any type of specialist for this condition?

If the tissue is persistent, occurs at a time other than the middle of normal puberty or if the tissue is large, your son may be sent to a pediatric endocrinologist (hormone doctor). A visit to an oncologist (cancer doctor), geneticist, or gastroenterologist (liver doctor) may also be needed if an underlying abnormality is found. A plastic surgeon can help with the removal of the breast tissue.

ELLEN S. SHER, MD
Endocrinology

BREATH-HOLDING SPELLS

Definition: Periods of holding breath.

Author's Comment: Witnessing your child holding his or her breath can be a frightening experience for parents, but the condition poses no serious threat for your child. It is important that you consult your child's doctor so that an accurate diagnosis can be established. These "spells" are age related and usually disappear by the time the child is five or six years old.

1. What is the cause of this condition?

Breath-holding spells are caused by instability of control of the blood flow to the brain in young children, usually set off by pain or an adverse emotional event.

2. How dangerous is this condition for my child, and what are the potential problems that can occur?

Even though this is a very scary-looking event, it should not cause problems. When they are older, these children do not have a higher chance of epilepsy or learning disabilities than the general population.

3. Is this condition a type of seizure?

No. This is not considered an epileptic seizure, since the brain is normal.

4. What diagnostic tests are needed to further define the cause or to rule out anything more serious?

A detailed history is most important. A complete blood count (CBC) should be done because of the association of iron deficiency anemia in some children with breath-holding spells. Sometimes an EKG, EEG, or a scan of the brain is needed, if there are unusual features in the history.

5. Will my child outgrow this condition and, if so, when?

This problem becomes less frequent after about two and a half years of age but can occur even up to six years old.

6. What is the best way to treat this condition if it occurs again?

Sometimes a spell can be averted by distracting the child when he or she is still crying hard, for example, by making a loud noise.

7. Do we need to see a neurologist or psychologist?

The pediatrician may send the child to a neurologist to help with the diagnosis. A psychologist can help if behavior issues are adding to the problems.

8. When do you wish to see my child again for this condition?

How often the child needs to be seen depends upon the severity of the problem. If the spells are infrequent, this may be handled just at routine wellness visits.

DAVID B. OWEN, MD
Neurology

BRONCHIOLITIS

Definition: A condition more common in infants that
                consists of an inflammation of the small
                airway passages and surrounding tissue
                leading to the lungs, causing cough,
                wheezing, and sometimes labored
                breathing.

Author's Comment: This respiratory illness can be a frightening condition for a parent to observe and to endure. It requires from the parent a great deal of vigilance and committed care. The parent needs to stay in close communication with the doctor and to know what signs to look for to determine whether the condition is getting worse.

1. What is the cause of this condition, and how did my child contract it?

Bronchiolitis is an infection of the lowest bronchioles in the respiratory tree caused by viral or bacterial infection. Children contract it from other individuals carrying the virus or bacteria. Depending on the age and medical condition of your child, he or she may be more susceptible to this type of illness.

Children under the age of three years (especially infants) and children that have other illnesses causing immunologic weakness usually contract bronchiolitis. Premature babies are at great risk and tend to have more serious bouts of bronchiolitis.

2. Is bronchiolitis contagious, and, if so, what measures should be taken to prevent its spread?

Yes, it is contagious and is passed via respiratory droplets. Caretakers should wash their hands after handling children with bronchiolitis, and sick children should be taught to cover their mouths when coughing. Nurses and doctors may wear protective gowns, gloves, and masks when caring for patients with bronchiolitis.

3. How is this condition treated?

Bronchiolitis is treated symptomatically. Most children can remain home when they have bronchiolitis and should only report to the doctor's office or emergency room when they have worsening respiratory distress. Hydration is of key importance when treating a child at home.

Over-the-counter cough medications do not usually help with the increased secretions or cough attacks. If a child is sick enough to go to the hospital, inhaled medications can sometimes help with the breathing difficulty. Premature babies sometimes qualify for monthly injections to prevent RSV bronchiolitis, which is a specific viral form of this illness. Talk to your pediatrician about this preventive measure if you feel your child may be eligible.

4. Are there medicines that can be useful during this illness?

Children with previously identified asthma may use their inhaled medicines to help with the cough of bronchiolitis. Otherwise, not many medications are useful during this illness.

5. How does the condition differ from asthma?

Asthma is a chronic condition, with exacerbations occurring repeatedly over time. Bronchiolitis is an infectious disease that affects children for one to four weeks. They both cause cough, but bronchiolitis may also have accompanying fever, runny nose, and rapid breathing patterns.

6. What are the danger signs that might indicate that the treatment is not progressing as well as it should?

Two things are important while your child suffers from bronchiolitis and eventually recovers. The first is hydration. If your child or baby cannot drink his or her necessary amount of liquid, you should contact your pediatrician. This is most easily tracked with wet diapers. A baby should have around six to eight wet diapers per day, and a child should urinate around four to five times per day. You can also assess hydration by the amount of saliva or moisture in the mouth. The other important assessment is of a child's breathing. If the chest is retracting so that the ribs are visible on inspiration and the abdomen is moving quickly, you should contact your pediatrician immediately for advice.

7. What complications can develop from this disorder?

The majority of children recover from bronchiolitis with no lasting symptoms. Even though the disease is vanishing, the cough can continue for up to four weeks. Some children may have more serious bouts of bronchiolitis requiring hospitalization, oxygen use, inhaled medications, or even intubation with mechanical ventilation. These cases are rare but can result in damaged lungs that require further medication for ease of breathing. These are the same medications used in children with asthma, and research now suggests that early bronchiolitis may be related to the development of asthma as a child.

8. Now that my child has had this condition, does it mean that it will occur over and over again?

Bronchiolitis tends to occur in children less than the age of five years. It is certainly normal to have the condition more than once, since many different viruses cause the mucous production and cough seen in bronchiolitis.

9. How long does it usually take for a child with this condition to show improvement?

Runny nose and fever usually only last for one to two weeks. The cough of bronchiolitis may persist past the initial phase, lasting as long as four weeks. Children are usually back to playing and full activity after two weeks of illness.

10. When do you wish to see my child again for follow-up of this disorder?

If your child is not improving after seven to ten days of cough, you should see your pediatrician again.

ANDREW S. GELFAND, MD
Pulmonary

BRONCHITIS

Definition: Infection of larger air tubes leading to the
lungs.

Author's Comment: What is frequently referred to as bronchitis in
childhood is generally a more diffused respiratory tract condition
involving more than just the bronchial tubes. Recurrent episodes of
this condition warrant a more thorough diagnostic workup.

1. What is the cause of this condition, and how did my child contract it?

Bronchitis is caused by viruses as well as some bacteria. It is
contracted by contact with other individuals carrying the virus or
bacteria. Typically, the particles are passed through respiratory
droplets. Bronchitis tends to occur in older children, after the age
that bronchiolitis occurs. This infection involves the trachea and
upper bronchi.

2. What are the complications that can occur from this condition?

The harsh cough associated with bronchitis can result in bloody secretions due to tearing of the respiratory mucosa. Vomiting may also occur due to cough or due to the presence of mucous in the stomach. Weakness in the immune system due to bronchitis may also cause other bacteria to invade the respiratory system, leading to pneumonia.

3. How is it treated?

If it is thought to be caused by bacteria, antibiotics may be prescribed. Sometimes medications to diminish the cough may be used, especially prior to bedtime. Inhaled medications may also help decrease the cough.

4. What are the potential side effects that can occur from the treatment?

Antibiotics can cause stomach upset in some patients. Some cough medicines cause drowsiness or sedation.

5. Is the condition contagious and, if so, for how long?

Yes, bronchitis is contagious. It typically lasts seven to ten days and is spread through respiratory droplets released during cough.

6. What restrictions should be placed on my child because of the condition?

Children should be instructed to cover their mouths when they cough and should wash their hands frequently. They should also limit their physical activity when noticing that they are panting or losing energy.

7. When can my child return to school and resume physical activity?

Your child can return to school and activity when there has been no fever for twenty-four hours, the cough has improved, and his or her energy level returns to near normal. This usually occurs after three to five days of illness.

8. What symptoms should I look for that would cause me to call you back again?

Signs that bronchitis is not resolving normally include a worsening in cough, increased mucous production, or a return of fever partially through the illness.

9. When do you wish to see my child again for this condition?

If you do not feel that your child is recovering normally from bronchitis, follow-up should be arranged.

ANDREW S. GELFAND, MD
Pulmonary

BRUISING
(Excessive)

Definition: A condition of areas of discoloration caused by superficial injury to the skin without laceration.

Author's Comment: Bruising on the legs is common in childhood and part of growing up. Bruising in widely distributed areas is more worrisome, and you should consult with your child's doctor for possible evaluation.

1. What causes this bruising?
Bruising is caused by bleeding into, or just under, the skin. Bruising below the knees is extremely common and is almost never a cause for concern. Unexplained bruising above the knees or on the chest, abdomen, or arms can be a cause for concern. Most bruising in children can be explained by injury, whether or not it was actually observed.

2. Is my child's bruising normal, or could there be an underlying problem in the blood?
If the child is showing significant, unexplained bruising, with or without nosebleeds, there might be a cause for concern. The physician

may order a number of tests to determine whether or not there is a condition in your child that may predispose the child to easy bruising.

3. Are any tests necessary to determine more specifically what is causing the bruising?

If a parent or physician suspects that the child is having excessive, unexplained bruising, then certain tests would be needed. Specifically, the doctor would order a platelet count. Platelets are little cells in the bloodstream that help the blood to clot. If there are insufficient platelets in the bloodstream, or if the platelets are not working well, this may result in easy, unexplained bruising. There are other tests the physician could order to determine whether or not the blood is too slow in clotting.

4. Would any vitamins or specific medicine be of help?

Supplemental vitamins are generally not helpful to prevent bruising that is either normal or abnormal. There are medicines that can be very helpful in treating problems such as low platelet count.

5. Do we need to consult with a hematologist (blood disorder specialist)?

If your pediatrician suspects that your child's bruising is abnormal and is due to a problem with blood clotting, or a problem with platelets, then the pediatrician would generally ask for a consultation with a pediatric hematologist.

6. Are there any danger signs I need to look for?

Yes. If your child is having unexplained bruising and this is accompanied by nosebleeding, mouth bleeding, or blood in the urine or stool, this should be brought to the attention of your child's physician immediately.

7. Do you need to see my child again regarding this condition?

In general, if abnormal bruising has been detected, then follow-up visits will be required.

CARL LENARSKY, MD

Hematology

CHICKEN POX
(Varicella)

Definition: An acute contagious infection with skin eruptions, fever, and various complaints of not feeling well.

Author's Comment: Thank heavens! The varicella vaccine has reduced the incidence of this disease considerably. Children contracting chickenpox in the general population are becoming fewer and fewer.

1. What causes this condition to occur?

Chickenpox is caused by a virus called varicella, which is related to other herpes viruses and is one of the most common infections of humans. The main symptoms are fever and a rash that looks like small blisters with clear fluid in them, occurring mainly on the arms, legs, and trunk, and somewhat less so on the face. The varicella vaccine has markedly reduced the occurrence of this disease in the past few years.

2. How long will my child be contagious, and how is it spread?

Your child will be contagious until all the skin lesions have crusted, although it is most contagious for the first few days. Chickenpox is spread by direct contact with an infected person, or occasionally by airborne spread from the respiratory secretions (coughing, etc.).

3. How long has my child been contagious prior to the appearance of the pox lesions?

A person with chickenpox is contagious from one to two days before the rash starts, until all the lesions have crusted over.

4. If another person was exposed to my child and contracted the disease, how long would it take for that person to eventually break out with the pox lesions?

It usually takes about fourteen to seventeen days after a person is exposed to chickenpox before he or she breaks out with chickenpox. This is called the incubation period. It can be as short as ten days or as long as twenty-one days.

5. If you have had this disease once, can you contract it again?

In almost all cases, if a person has had chickenpox once, he or she will not come down with the disease again. This is called being immune to the disease. For most people, immunity to chickenpox is lifelong. There are exceptions, though. People whose immune systems become impaired can get chickenpox again. And another, milder form of the infection, called zoster, or shingles, can develop many years after the initial infection. Shingles is usually limited to one part of the body, like a strip along the back, if it does occur. Most people, however, never get shingles or any other form of chickenpox after their initial infection with the chickenpox virus.

6. How is it treated and for how long?

Usually, chickenpox is not treated. It runs its course in several days. Your doctor may recommend an antiviral drug called acyclovir, or a related medicine, in some circumstances. These medicines are especially helpful in persons with immune problems.

7. What complications can occur as a result of this disease?

Most children with chickenpox have no complications. If complications occur, it is most likely to be a secondary infection of the skin lesions with strep or staph bacteria and may require an antibiotic. Other less common complications include pneumonia, encephalitis, Reye syndrome (which can be prevented by avoiding aspirin-containing medicines during the chickenpox illness), and bleeding under the skin at the site of the lesions, all of which are uncommon in people with normal immune systems.

8. Is there any way to shorten its course?

The antiviral medicines like acyclovir can shorten the course by a day or so, if they are started within the first day of the illness.

9. Will it leave any permanent scars?

The chickenpox will almost always resolve without any scarring unless the lesions become infected with a bacteria, which is more likely if the child picks at the lesions.

10. Is there any way to prevent a person exposed to my child from coming down with the disease?

The chickenpox vaccine can be given up to three days or so after an exposure and still protect a person from developing the disease, although it is less than 100 percent effective. Even if it does not prevent the disease entirely, it will usually make the disease more mild.

11. What kind of follow-up is needed?

None, unless your child seems to be developing a complication, such as very high fevers, infection of a lesion (increased redness or pus oozing from a lesion), trouble breathing, or change in mental status (incoherence, lethargy, etc).

GREGORY R. ISTRE, MD
Infectious Diseases

COLIC

Definition: **Pronounced irritability in the first months of life.**

Author's Comment: This condition can cause moms to feel helpless and depressed. I have always felt the best way for moms to get through this difficult period is for them to stay in close contact with their pediatrician and to have the infant checked and rechecked for reassurance.

1. What causes colic?

There is no general agreement as to what colic is. Crying for three hours a day for three or more days per week for greater than three weeks in a healthy infant usually defines a "colicky infant." Most doctors believe that colic may be the result of a variety of developmental immaturities in the infant's gastrointestinal tract. The symptoms may be secondary to immaturity of digestive enzymes, gut immunity, absorption, motility (the colon's ability to contract), or any combination thereof.

2. How long is it supposed to last?

Most infants will have symptoms from birth to about three months. A rare child may have symptoms up to nine months of age.

3. Is there anything in a breastfeeding mother's diet that might contribute to the colic?

In some infants, having the mother avoid caffeine, spicy foods, or foods containing cow's milk protein may be beneficial. Having the child empty a complete breast per feeding may give the child the richer "hindmilk," leaving the infant more satisfied after nursing.

4. With a baby that is formula fed, does changing the formula to a soy or possibly a protein hydrolysate help?

If the child is experiencing irritability from a protein intolerance, then a change to a different protein source may be helpful. Soy may be attempted first. If the child is still having problems after three to five days, then a change to a hydrolysate formula may be beneficial.

5. What about medicines—do they help?

There have not been any reproducible studies that demonstrate any benefit from medications for true colic. The inability to find a "universal treatment" is likely the result of the variety of possible causes for colic (as outlined earlier) and the nonspecific nature of the symptoms between different infants.

6. Is there anything else that a parent can do to make the child feel better?

Symptomatic, soothing maneuvers may be beneficial. Sometimes a warm bath, wrapping in a soft blanket, a ride in the car, a gentle rocking motion, or soft sounds may help. Making certain that caretakers are as relaxed and not stressed as possible is important as well: "taking turns" with the crying child may also help diffuse the stressful situation.

7. How long should I let my baby cry, and does crying over a period of time harm the baby in any way?

Crying does not harm the baby. The acceptable duration of crying depends on multiple factors, such as the child's usual trend for fussiness, parental stress levels, and even cultural considerations. If the child is vigorous, eating, thriving, with good color, and without a fever, then periods up to thirty minutes or more would not be unusual. Sometimes giving the child breaks from the interventions listed earlier for five to ten minutes may be beneficial to allow the child to self-soothe without parental or environmental overstimulation.

8. Are any tests needed to make sure that the baby's irritability is nothing more serious than colic?

In most instances of infantile colic, tests are not necessary. An evaluation by your pediatrician can determine if any are in order. A stool sample to check for rectal bleeding can help determine if milk protein allergies are involved. Sometimes, your pediatrician may order an upper GI X ray series or abdominal sonogram to exclude gastrointestinal or renal anatomical defects as the cause for the irritability.

9. What signs or symptoms do I look for that would make me need to call you back?

Most infants with colic have a usual, predictable pattern of crying, typically at the same times of the day. If the crying is prolonged or not in keeping with the child's usual behavior, then an assessment by your physician may be warranted. Lethargy, fever, pallor, feeding refusal, excessive vomiting, unusual constipation or diarrhea, or rectal bleeding may require further assessment.

10. When do you want to see my child again for this condition?

If none of the above conditions apply, then reassessment for colic may be necessary if the symptoms persist beyond three to four months of age.

KENDALL O. BROWN, MD
Gastroenterology

CONSTIPATION

Definition: Infrequency of bowel movements.

Author's Comment: This is a very common cause for parents to seek advice from the doctor. Once constipation persists for awhile, it can be self-perpetuating and can cause a great deal of concern in the family. Fortunately, there are effective ways of treating this condition at every age.

1. What causes this condition to occur in my child?

Constipation is a very common childhood complaint. Few cases of constipation are the result of serious underlying diseases. Most have no organic or physical cause. Constipation most likely results from a combination of diet, environment, and behavior, along with intrinsic tendencies of the colon with regard to water reabsorption and the colon's ability to contract (motility).

2. What are the potential problems that can arise from this condition?

The most common complaint is pain, which may lead to withholding behavior as a result of passing large, hard stools. This may result in further constipation (fecal impaction) and soiling. Some children will have streaks of blood in their feces from rectal or anal tears. Some might be difficult to toilet train for stool but able to train for urine. Soiling occurs when more liquid stool from higher up seeps around a retained hard mass of stool that has become "stuck" in a dilated rectum. In more advanced cases, the child may have a distended abdomen, loss of appetite, and weight loss.

3. How is it treated?

Treatment includes evacuating an impaction or blockage of retained stool (if present), softening to eliminate the pain and discomfort associated with the process, addressing issues related to family dynamics and toilet training, and dietary modifications.

Management depends upon the patient's age, duration of symptoms, behavior, and past experience with various regimens. In infants and small children, adding high content, poorly digestible sugars such as corn sweetener (Karo syrup) or undiluted fruit juice (apple, pear, or prune) to the diet may be useful.

In older children, lubricating agents (mineral oil) or osmotic laxatives such as milk of magnesia or polyethelene glycol (Miralax or Glycolax) are useful. Stimulant laxatives containing senna, cascara, or phenolphthalein should be avoided in children. Consult your child's physician to determine which regimen or medication would be most appropriate.

4. What are the potential side effects from the treatment?

Most current recommended therapies for constipation are safe. Again, habit-forming, stimulating laxatives should be avoided. Enemas and suppositories should be used under physician supervision to prevent adverse effects and to avoid further negative behavior resulting from rectal pain.

5. Can diet play a role in the cause and/or treatment of constipation?

In most cases, there is no clear association between diet and constipation. A low-residue, high-fat, high-calcium diet with limited nondigestible fiber and ample water is frequently seen in constipated children between one to two years of age.

Reducing high-fat meals, cheese, and perhaps excessive cow's milk may help uncomplicated constipation, but this should not be so restrictive as to limit adequate caloric intake. High-fiber diets are usually of little benefit because they are not well received by preschool children, are generally not effective in achieving consistent long-term stool softening, and do little to address recurrent impaction and soiling.

6. What further diagnostic tests are needed?

In most cases, no testing is required for childhood constipation.

7. If the constipation is chronic, does my child need to see a gastrointestinal specialist?

Referral to a pediatric gastroenterologist should be considered for recurrent impaction, abdominal swelling, growth failure, urinary symptoms, or prior treatment failures. Long-standing constipation from infancy, failure to pass meconium (first stool) in the first days of life, or developmental delays also merit further evaluation.

8. What symptoms would cause me to call you back regarding this condition?

Inform your doctor when your child has severe abdominal pain, no stool output for three to five days, constant soiling not responding to therapy, abdominal swelling, vomiting, refusal to eat, marked rectal bleeding, urinary incontinence, and/or painful urination.

9. What kind of follow-up is needed in the future?

Most cases will gradually resolve over time with the combination of appropriate medications, intervention for withholding behavior, and toilet training. Periodic visits should be scheduled until the problem resolves.

KENDALL O. BROWN, MD
Gastroenterology

CORNEAL ABRASION

Definition: A scratch on the clear front surface of the eye (cornea).

Author's Comment: This is a potentially serious occurrence and warrants close follow-up with your child's physician. Fortunately, this condition usually heals in forty-eight to seventy-two hours.

1. What actually has happened to my child's eye?

The transparent covering on the front surface of the eye is called the cornea. When the front surface of the cornea (epithelium) is removed by a direct contact injury, a corneal abrasion occurs. This injury will usually cause pain, light sensitivity, tearing, and swelling. It also may feel as if there is something in the eye.

2. What potential dangers does this condition pose?

Infection may occur, especially if the injury was from a "dirty" object such as a fingernail or tree branch, and vision may be impaired due to the resulting development of a cloudy cornea.

Vision may also be affected by surface irregularities in the cornea at the site of the injury.

3. How is it treated and for how long?

Treatment of corneal abrasions includes the use of antibiotic drops or ointment and a tight patch over the eye for twenty-four to forty-eight hours. Depending on the size of the abrasion, healing usually occurs within twenty-four hours. Antibiotic drops or ointment are continued for several days after the abrasion has healed.

4. Are there any side effects that can occur from treatment?

Corneal abrasions may heal inadequately, particularly if the abrasion is irregular. If the new surface does not stick down sufficiently to the injured area, weeks or months later a spontaneous corneal abrasion may occur. This may occur at night or early in the morning with characteristic eye pain. Lubricating the eye with ointment before bedtime for several weeks after the initial injury may help to avoid this complication. Steroid drops should not be used at the onset for treatment of corneal abrasions since they may delay wound healing and increase the possibility of infection. Anesthetic eye drops to dull the pain should also be avoided because they will also slow down healing.

5. Do we need to see an ophthalmologist (eye specialist) and, if so, when?

If your pediatrician feels that the corneal abrasion is not healing in a timely fashion or he suspects a more serious injury or infection, he may refer you to an ophthalmologist for further evaluation.

6. When do you wish to see my child again in the future for this condition?

Your child should be checked within twenty-four to forty-eight hours of the injury to make sure that proper healing of the cornea is taking place and there are no signs of infection. Any signs of increased light sensitivity, tearing, or pain in the previously injured eye should warrant a visit to your pediatrician or ophthalmologist.

JOEL LEFFLER, MD
Ophthalmology

CRADLE CAP
(Seborrheic Dermatitis)

Definition: Inflammation and scaliness of the scalp and surrounding area.

Author's Comment: This is a very common condition in infancy and is relatively easy to treat. It may be confused with the more chronic condition of infantile eczema.

1. What causes this condition, and how did my child develop it?

The cause of seborrheic dermatitis is unknown.

2. How long will it last?

The scaling is most noticeable during the first four to six weeks of life. It usually clears up within a few months but can occasionally last up to one year of age.

3. How does it differ from dandruff?

Seborrheic dermatitis of the scalp in babies is called cradle cap; in teenagers and adults it is called dandruff. It is the same condition, but the infant form tends to have a thick, yellowish "stuck-on" type of scale, whereas the adult form has white, flaky scale. The treatment of these two forms is the same.

4. How does it differ from eczema (atopic dermatitis) of the scalp?

These two conditions are both pink and scaly and can look very similar. Both conditions can also involve the skin on the arms, legs, and trunk. The scale of seborrheic dermatitis tends to be thicker and yellowish and often goes away at a few months of age. It is not usually itchy and may involve the diaper area. It also commonly causes red moist skin lesions in the creases of the underarms, neck, and groin.

Eczema has a fine flaky scale, is very itchy, and tends to last longer (years, rather than months). Signs that a baby is itchy include fussiness, poor sleep, scratching, or rubbing his or her head on the mattress. Eczema in the diaper area is uncommon.

5. Can cradle cap get infected?

It is uncommon for seborrheic dermatitis to get infected, but it does happen occasionally. Skin infection is much more common with eczema.

6. What is the treatment?

If it is mild, no treatment may be needed. For thick scale, gently massaging baby or mineral oil into the scalp helps soften the scale. The scale can then be removed gently with a soft hairbrush. Dandruff shampoos used daily or every other day can also be helpful.

7. Are there side effects of the treatment that can be anticipated, and how long does it take to get better?

Improvement is usually noted within a few days to a week after starting treatment. As long as the shampoo is kept out of the baby's eyes, there are very few side effects. Dandruff shampoos can cause some dryness of the hair or mild skin irritation, especially if there is an open cut or scratch on the scalp.

8. What signs do I look for to call you back?

If your child is not improving at all after a week or so, or if he or she shows signs of persistent itching, then you should call back.

9. When do you wish to see my child again for this condition?

Since cradle cap is a temporary and harmless condition, no follow-up visit is needed unless your child seems to be getting worse rather than better. Although, if your child develops red, flat-topped, scab-like bumps within the scaly, pink areas of skin, particularly in the skin folds of the groin, underarms, or behind the ears, then your child should be reevaluated, as this may be a sign of an uncommon but more serious condition called histiocytosis.

K. ROBIN CARDER, MD
Dermatology

CRANIOSYNOSTOSIS

Definition: Premature closure of the cranial sutures (growth centers that occur between the bones in the skull) usually resulting in some cosmetic deformity.

Author's Comment: Adults with oddly shaped skulls may have this condition.

1. What caused this condition to occur in my child?

Craniosynostosis is a congenital deformity of the skull that is present at birth but may not become apparent until after delivery for some time. When looking in retrospect, the deformity is often seen in early pictures from the day of delivery or soon thereafter.

It occurs when one or more of the cranial sutures (joints between skull bones) closes prematurely. The shape of the deformity is specific to the affected structure. Craniosynostosis may also be part of a larger syndromal deformity that affects other areas like the skin, facial development, hands, and feet. These cases are usually more severe.

The majority of craniosynostosis deformities are the result of a developmental anomaly in the genetic code, most of which have not been isolated. However, the cause of some specific types has been isolated in the genetic code and is known to be passed down from generation to generation. There have been no identifiable risk factors related to the parents or the maternal prenatal care.

It is important to note that, besides cosmetic deformities, there can be significant developmental issues that need to be addressed with this condition.

2. Is there a genetic link?

There is a genetic link to many of the craniosynostoses. Not all the genetic code anomalies have been located yet.

3. What diagnostic tests are needed to further define this condition or its impact on my child's brain?

Most cases can be diagnosed by the physical exam and medical history. However, this is only a deformity in the shape of the skull; it does not apply to anything below the skull, such as the brain. Additional evaluations of the skull deformity can be obtained with X rays of the skull. If there is some concern about the brain development, a CT scan is warranted.

Many experts also advocate developmental examinations for children with craniosynostosis. These examinations need to be done over time, so that the effects can be measured as the child develops. Developmental examinations are often performed before and after surgical correction so that any delay can be diagnosed and treated as soon as possible.

Other examinations can be performed by a medical anthropologist. This type of specialist measures multiple sites on the skull to gain information on the development and asymmetries of the deformity. It is a very good, noninvasive way to assess the skull deformity.

4. What is the treatment for this condition, and when do we need to see a craniofacial surgeon (a plastic surgeon who specializes in this type of disorder)?

It is important to seek out a specialist craniofacial surgeon when you or the pediatrician suspect the diagnosis of craniosynostosis. The treatment for craniosynostosis is surgical (no amount of physical therapy or helmet therapy can achieve correction because the sutures are closed). The surgery involves the combined talents of a craniofacial surgeon and pediatric neurosurgeon. In addition, the child should be cared for at a craniofacial center that specializes in the care and treatment of children with complex craniofacial problems.

The surgery itself involves the removal and then the reshaping of the skull, called remodeling. This is done through an incision across the width of the scalp to gain access to the skull and the abnormal suture. Once the skull has been reshaped and the bones replaced (either with dissolvable sutures or dissolvable plates and screws), the scalp is closed, most often with dissolvable sutures.

Recently, there is a move to correct these skull deformities with less invasive techniques. These can be performed via smaller access incisions, instruments with lights and cameras (sometimes but not always necessary), and postoperative helmet therapy. This type of operation is controversial in some centers, but the research is currently identifying the best cases for this approach. It is important that surgeons be trained in both types of techniques as often the minimally invasive techniques may not be warranted in your child.

5. What are the complications of the treatment, and what kind of cosmetic results can we expect?

Surgery is never without risks. These risks, however, can be kept to a minimum when the treating physicians and the center specialize in this type of treatment. Craniofacial centers are the most popular places where these procedures are performed.

The risks include (but are not limited to) bleeding, infection, poor bone coverage, brain damage, seizures, stroke, and death. These are severe risks but are significantly limited at these centers. Children may require blood transfusions, but this risk decreases with the age at the time of the operation.

Surgery may be performed from six weeks of age to one year depending on the diagnosis and severity of the deformity. The expected results are most often excellent. Many children may have some asymmetries immediately after surgery but over time, they tend to go away with continued, normal skull growth.

6. Left untreated, what would be the likely outcome?

The majority of craniosynostotic deformities, if left untreated, would result in a persistent craniofacial deformity with the skull deformity often leading to a facial deformity. It is important to understand that when the sutures close, they affect not only the skull but also the face.

Some of the deformities are very mild and may not present an aesthetic or functional problem. These types of early suture closure can be watched and possibly left untreated without harmful effects on the child.

7. What kind of follow-up will be needed for this condition, and when do you wish to see my child again?

Follow-up for these children is uniform. The children are seen at an initial visit to the specialist, then before surgery for a preoperative evaluation, and then again postoperatively at two to three weeks.

After the postoperative visit, the follow-up becomes a bit looser depending on the distance the family has to travel. A typical schedule will be at three months postoperatively, one year and then yearly until the age of twelve to thirteen. In some cases, more frequent follow-up may be necessary.

It is important for the children to be seen by the entire team at these yearly visits. The team may include the medical anthropologist (for head measurements), developmental pediatrician or psychologist, social worker, speech therapist, and others. These evaluations often require a full-day visit. Depending on the growth and development of the child, further investigative evaluations may be necessary, including CT scan or an MRI (magnetic resonance imaging) to evaluate brain development.

DAVID GENECOV, MD
Craniofacial Surgery

CROHN'S DISEASE
(Regional Ileitis)

Definition: Inflammation primarily of the small intestine with resultant fever, diarrhea, and weight loss.

Author's Comment: This chronic intestinal condition can cause children hours of misery. However, it can be adequately treated by doctors who are well schooled in the medicinal treatment of this disorder. Usually, children can function normally despite this condition.

1. What causes this disorder, and how did my child contract it?

The cause of Crohn's disease is unknown at this time. Some people are genetically predisposed to develop Crohn's disease.

2. What is the natural course of this disease over a long period of time?

The natural course of the disease is unpredictable fluctuations in disease symptoms with eventual worsening of disease if not treated.

3. Is the disorder hereditary, or are there environmental factors involved?

The disease is partially hereditary with environmental or biologic triggers. The environmental and biologic triggers are being studied at this time.

4. Does diet play a role?

Diet may play a role in causing or exacerbating symptoms. However, after a person is diagnosed with Crohn's disease, there are no restrictions on his or her diet unless specific food groups are known to exacerbate symptoms in a particular patient.

5. What medicines are used to treat my child's disorder, and how long are they to be used?

Typical medications include mesalamine, prednisone, azathioprine, antibiotics as well as other newer anti-inflammatory drugs. Length of therapy will depend on the medication used as well as severity of symptoms.

6. How soon do the medicines take effect, and when will my child start getting better?

Medications usually take effect within a few days, and your child should start feeling better in a few days. Azathioprine may take up to two months before it has any effect.

7. What are the potential side effects of the medicines?

Each of the medications can have differing side effects, but many of the side effects weaken the patient's immune system. Other typical side effects may include rash, diarrhea, headache, and muscle aches. Low blood count is a serious side effect that is monitored.

8. Does surgery play a role in the treatment now or later on?

Surgery does play a role in Crohn's disease. Surgery is considered if there is an obstruction in the gastrointestinal tract or if medications cannot adequately control symptoms. However, surgery does not control the disease, unlike in ulcerative colitis, which is another form of inflammatory bowel disease seen in children.

9. What signs do I look for to determine whether my child is getting worse?

Typical signs of worsening disease include severe abdominal pain, increasing diarrhea, unexplained fever, or weight loss.

10. Do I need to see a pediatric gastroenterologist?

A pediatric gastroenterologist is often helpful in monitoring your child's symptoms and treating the disease, but it is up to your pediatrician to determine if a gastroenterologist's expertise is needed.

11. What symptoms would warrant my calling you back?

Call back if there are any concerning symptoms, such as persistent abdominal pain, diarrhea, or unexplained fever.

12. How often do you wish to see my child regarding this condition?

Your child will be seen by the pediatrician often in conjunction with the pediatric gastroenterologist in a team effort to control symptoms.

The frequency of visits will be determined by the severity of the symptoms as well as response to medications.

JACK AN, MD
Gastroenterology

CROUP

Definition: Inflammation of the larynx resulting in a barking type cough.

Author's Comment: This is, at times, a frightening disease for parents, as they witness their child struggling to breathe. It requires a great deal of parental vigilance with close medical supervision. Though it may be a grueling period of time, the condition is usually much improved in two to three days. Nonetheless, once you have experienced this condition, you will never forget the sound of the high-pitched barking cough that your child displayed.

1. What causes this condition, and how did my child contract it?

Croup occurs in two forms, infectious and noninfectious. The infectious type is caused by one of many viruses, most famously the parainfluenza species. This virus is passed via respiratory droplets, as are many upper respiratory viral infections. The noninfectious type is also known as "spasmodic" croup. This type of cough can recur in some children and might be related to allergies.

Gastroesophageal reflux (GER) may also contribute to a croupy cough.

Croup is characterized by a barky cough and stridor, which is noisy, high-pitched breathing, especially while breathing inward. These symptoms are caused by inflammation of the trachea and larynx. Symptoms are usually much worse in the evenings and nighttime.

2. Is it contagious and for how long?

Yes, croup is contagious. Prior to the typical barky cough and stridor, children frequently have fever and runny nose. Symptoms can last for three to five days, and children are most likely contagious during the entire illness.

3. What can be done to treat it?

Home therapies for croup involve changes in the temperature of the air being breathed. Some parents can take their child outside into the cool night air for relief, and others run a hot shower in a closed bathroom to create warm vapor. Medicinal treatment for the barky cough or stridor can include inhaled anti-inflammatories such as epinephrine or steroids.

4. Are antibiotics or steroids effective as part of the treatment, and, if so, how long should they be used?

Antibiotics are not helpful, since croup is caused by viruses. Steroids have been shown to decrease the airway inflammation. Most commonly, children will receive either a single injection of dexamethasone (Decadron) or one oral dose of this medication. This form of steroid remains in the body for around three days, and thus only one dose is necessary. Inhaled steroids have also been shown to help and can be used twice a day for three to four days.

5. If used, what are the potential side effects from these medicines?

Since the steroids are used sparingly, side effects are greatly diminished. Most often blood sugar values will increase, so children with diabetes should be extra careful. Vomiting or an upset stomach can also occur with the oral medication. Occasionally, children can become more emotional.

6. Are steroids effective in the treatment?

Yes, steroids can decrease the inflammation present in the airway. This means that the cough and difficulty breathing may be lessened. However, steroids do not affect the overall illness, so fever, fussiness, nasal discharge, and sleep changes will still be present.

7. What are the potential complications of croup, and how will I recognize them?

Inflammation of the airway causes the loud cough and difficulty breathing seen in croup. Complications surround the difficulty breathing, and can include mild-to-severe respiratory distress, difficulty controlling secretions (saliva and mucous), or difficulty eating and drinking (which can lead to dehydration).

You will recognize complications by the amount of work your child has to do to breathe. This work of breathing is known as retractions (using accessory muscle in the neck, ribs, and/or stomach to help with breathing). Sometimes nasal flaring and grunting can also occur.

8. What am I supposed to do if I encounter these complications?

If you feel that your child's breathing is worsening, you should call your pediatrician and report to the nearest emergency room for evaluation. Try to keep your child calm, as breathing always sounds worse when a child is screaming or crying.

9. Are there any specific precautions I should take in regard to my child's sleeping?

Typically, breathing becomes less labored when a child falls asleep. A humidifier may also provide some comfort in a child with croup.

10. Should I sleep in the same room?

If you feel more comfortable sleeping in the same room, this may give both the parent and child an easier night.

11. How long will it take for my child to show improvement?

Most viruses run their course in seven to ten days. The fever and runny nose may precede the croupy cough by two to three days, and the stridor usually lasts three to four days.

12. When should I call you back again?

If you do not see improvement in your child after one week, you should call your pediatrician. Close contact with the pediatrician's office during the illness can provide you both guidance and reassurance.

13.   When do you wish to see my child again regarding this condition?

If your child recovers from the croupy cough and stridor after three to four days, there is no need for a follow-up visit. If you do not feel that the cough has changed or that the illness is somehow different from the typical croup description, you should see your pediatrician. If your child has croup more than once, you should call your doctor as well.

TIMOTHY TRONE, MD
Otolaryngology

CUTS
(Requiring Stitches)

Author's Comment: Some cuts that required stitches by doctors in the past are now glued. Be sure to make your house as safe as possible; coffee tables and fireplace hearths are still prime offenders.

1. Will stitches be required to repair this cut?

Usually, cuts that tend to gape and you can see tissue (fat or muscle) underneath will require some form of closure. Currently many small cuts require only surgical glue, though cuts on the face (especially in the eyebrow region) should still be sutured. The decision to close a cut with sutures is usually made by the physician and is based on the size and depth of the cut, its location, and the probability that there will be tension on the repair site.

2. Are there any treatment options available other than stitching?

Steri-strip band-aids and butterfly band-aids can be used on very small cuts, though surgical glue is the most preferred option. Sometimes surgical staples are used, especially in scalp wounds.

3. When is a cut serious enough to require a surgeon or plastic surgeon?

In children, many parents prefer a plastic surgeon for injuries to the face, especially the lips, ears, and nose. For simple lacerations most physicians comfortable with suturing small lacerations can be trusted. For deep lacerations, lacerations where there is continued bleeding; lacerations from animal bites; or lacerations where there may be glass, wood, or metal, a surgeon should be consulted. In these cases, repair in the operating room may be necessary.

4. Will the cut leave a scar? If so, what can be done to minimize the scarring?

All cuts will leave a scar that fades with time. The appearance of the scar is lessened with appropriate repair of the laceration with minimal tension on the skin edges. Applying vitamin E to a wound may also help reduce scarring. There are many over-the-counter remedies that may be of benefit though none can provide any true scientific proof that one is better than the other. It is important to keep scars protected against sunburn for the first year after a cut since a scar will burn more easily. As a result, the scar will "tattoo" darker than the surrounding skin.

5. Are the stitches absorbable? If not, when do the stitches need to be taken out?

Some sutures dissolve on their own and do not need to be removed. Ask your doctor if he has used these kind of sutures. If no, most stitches on the face should come out in three to five days. Otherwise, sutures are usually removed at one week.

6. What signs do I look for that might indicate that the cut is getting infected?

Signs that a wound is getting infected include increased pain, redness, or swelling around the wound, red tracks going away from the wound, increased warmth of the wound, and drainage from the cut. Signs like fever and marked swelling indicate a possible severe infection. If any of these signs develop, you should call your doctor immediately.

7. Should I leave the cut open or covered, and will it need a topical antibiotic?

Most cuts should be covered for at least two days, if possible; in some areas this is not possible, especially on the lips or on the scalp.

8. What do I do to prevent my child from pulling out the stitches?

Fortunately, most children will not pull out their own stitches because it hurts to pull on them.

9. What physical limitations should I impose to protect the cut and for how long?

Most children should be kept out of sports and physical education classes for at least two to three weeks because bumping the incision can reopen the cut. Also, the incision should be kept dry for at least two to three days.

10. Does my child need a tetanus shot as a result of the cut?

If your child is up-to-date on his or her tetanus immunizations, a tetanus booster is rarely needed. In certain instances where the child is due for immunizations soon or there is gross contamination of the cut, a tetanus booster may be given.

11. When do you wish to see my child again to remove the stitches?

Stitches should be removed from cuts to the face and neck at three days unless your physician tells you otherwise. For most other lacerations, stitches are removed in seven days. If the wound is extensive or there is excessive tension on the wound, stitches are sometimes left in for a longer period of time.

KEVIN M. KADESKY, MD
Surgery

DEVELOPMENTAL DELAY

Definition: **A delay in the area of physical or mental development.**

Author's Comment: If you or your physician suspect a developmental delay in your child, there are public-sponsored agencies in most states that will evaluate and provide treatment for these conditions at a very young age. Early intervention is most important in addressing cognitive or motor areas of questionable delay.

1. What is the cause of this condition in my child?

A child may be at risk for developmental delay as a result of biological or environmental factors, or both. Certain prenatal conditions related to maternal or fetal health may predispose a child to slow development. Problems at birth, including prematurity, may adversely affect the pace of development. These conditions are usually obvious soon after delivery. Metabolic issues, birth defects, and feeding problems are a few examples.

Environmental issues in infancy and toddlerhood may influence development and are usually associated with families with social risk factors. Medical illness may interfere with a child's exploration of the environment. Hospitalization and the child's response to it can cause regression or slow progress in development. Similar conditions in the family, such as late talking, may attribute to a child's delays as well.

2. What kind of treatment is necessary, and how long will it take to see improvement?

Your child may be referred for specialized therapeutic intervention if the delay is greater than 25 percent. Depending on the issues, speech and language, physical, or occupational therapy may be recommended. If delays are less severe, a good preschool program may be helpful. Medication is rarely recommended, unless behavior problems interfere with a child's ability to benefit from therapy. Progress in therapy can be variable, but a minimum of six weeks is usually necessary to measure progress in therapy.

3. What are the chances that, with treatment, these delays can be overcome and what can we expect for long-term results?

Children with developmental delays have a wide variety of abilities and it is difficult to make generalizations. Not every child with a delay will "catch up" to his or her chronologic age in development. It has been shown that children who receive early intervention services make more progress, and the effects are long-lasting. Measuring a child's progress over time gives a better idea of whether catch-up development is occurring. Periodic reassessment by your child's therapist is the best way to view results over the long term and to give you an idea of what to expect in the future.

4. How much of a difference would it make if no treatment at all took place?

It would be difficult to estimate a child's progress with or without therapy because each child is unique and brings his or her own set of abilities and challenges to therapy. In general, a child's drive to develop is innate. Letting the child develop at his or her own pace, with the set of biological and environmental factors the child possesses, is certainly an option. However, the rapid development that occurs during a child's first five years of life suggests that it is reasonable to begin therapy while the rapid brain growth is occurring.

Your child's early experiences have an impact on his or her pace of development, and early intervention provides services to help advance to the next stage. Parents are guided to help their children along the developmental continuum with the assistance of the therapist who is specially trained in child development. The pace of progress may be much slower without this assistance.

5. Does my child need to be evaluated by a neurologist or a developmental specialist?

Your pediatrician will perform a general medical evaluation and help you determine if this is necessary. In general, a child with a mild-to-moderate developmental delay in one area probably does not need a referral to a specialist. If there is more than one stream of development affected, it is usually an indication for further evaluation.

If there are concerns about unusual movements or neurologic findings are present on physical exam, a neurology referral is warranted. If concerns center around a child's cognitive, speech, or overall development, you may be referred to a developmental specialist. If the child has birth defects or there is a prominent family history of developmental issues, a genetic evaluation may be helpful.

6. What kind of follow-up will be needed with you in the future for this condition?

Periodic follow-up for developmental issues is important. Once your child is receiving intervention services, periodic reassessment will be provided by the therapist. Ongoing surveillance of overall development will be provided by your pediatrician. Monitoring other streams of behavior and development is important to detect other issues as they arise. This is usually done in the course of routine pediatric care, at your annual health evaluation.

LISA W. GENECOV, MD
Developmental Disorders

DIABETES (Mellitus)

Definition: A disorder of carbohydrate metabolism resulting from a deficiency of insulin production in the pancreas or a resistance to insulin giving rise to an elevated blood sugar.

Author's Comment: This condition can be adequately regulated by good medical supervision with diligence to daily medication monitoring, blood sugar monitoring, and adherence to consistent dietary principles. Diabetic summer camps can provide not only recreation but also diabetic education as well as a sense of camaraderie with kids that have the same disorder.

1. What causes this condition, and how did my child contract it?

A distinction should be made between Type 1 and Type 2 diabetes. Type 1 is caused by an autoimmune process whereby the body identifies the insulin-producing cells in the pancreas as foreign and produces antibodies to destroy the cells. After about 90 percent of the cells are destroyed, symptoms of urinary frequency, excessive thirst and weight loss occur. We do not know why some people's bodies identify the pancreas cells as foreign, although there is a genetic component. No studies have demonstrated that a particular diet or lifestyle determines who will get Type 1 diabetes.

In contrast, Type 2 diabetes is caused by a resistance to insulin, and consequently insulin levels may be high. Type 2 diabetes has a strong genetic component, and the development of this disorder is clearly related to obesity, dietary excesses, and sedentary lifestyle.

2. What is the normal course of the disease, and where do I go for more education?

Without treatment, both types of diabetes follow an unremitting course. Initially, the symptoms may be limited to urinary frequency and excess thirst but will progress to more serious problems. Generally, the course of untreated Type 1 diabetes is rapid. Most children experience about two weeks of urinary symptoms and thirst that is then followed by weight loss and fatigue and finally progressive somnolence (drowsiness), respiratory difficulties, and shock.

Type 2 tends to follow a more slowly developing course and may be present for months without significant symptoms, but without treatment the condition will eventually result in organ damage. Your pediatrician can give you more information, but if your child be diagnosed with diabetes, he or she should be cared for by a pediatric endocrinologist (diabetes specialist) in a multidisciplinary clinic where educating you and your child is a priority.

3. What medicines are used for treatment, and are there any potential side effects as a result of their usage?

Insulin injections are used to replace the insulin that the body does not make in Type 1 diabetes. The amount of insulin used is dependent on anticipated dietary intake and amount of physical activity. Obviously, this can be difficult to plan and predict, and the most serious side effect of insulin is to drop the blood sugar too low. This can cause seizure or loss of consciousness. It is crucial to monitor the blood sugar with a child on insulin and always have glucose gel and injectable glucagon on hand in case of a reaction. Other side effects of insulin include hypertrophy (swelling) of fat cells at injection sites and minimal discomfort of the injections.

Medications used to treat Type 2 diabetes include oral pills that make the body produce more insulin and/or pills that make the body more sensitive to the insulin already produced. Sometimes patients with Type 2 diabetes need insulin injections as well.

4. What is the best way to regulate the dosage of the medication?

Frequent monitoring of blood sugar is key. In addition, because blood sugar is influenced by food and activity, behavioral consistency can help determine rational dose changes.

5. How big a role does diet play in the control and progression of the disease?

With Type 1 diabetes, consistency in diet helps you and your physician calculate rational insulin dosing. With more experience, many children and their families have learned how to modify the doses at certain times to allow more food freedom. With Type 2 diabetes, weight control and increasing activity can significantly improve the progression of the disease, and these are a mainstay of treatment.

6. What signs do I look for to know if my child is getting in trouble with the disease?

Among the worrisome signs are any changes in your child's level of alertness, vomiting, rapid breathing, fruity smelling breath, or even increasing difficulty with urinary frequency or excess thirst. However, this list is not exhaustive, and therefore any unusual symptom should be promptly brought to your doctor's attention.

7. Do we need to see an endocrinologist (diabetes specialist)?

Yes. Diabetes can be a difficult disorder to control and an endocrinologist has the medical training in the treatment of this specific disorder, as well as the information to educate and empower both you and your child to best manage the illness.

8. Do my other children need to be tested for diabetes?

With Type 2 diabetes, because there is a strong genetic predisposition, healthy eating habits and adequate exercise should be instituted for all family members. Any child who is symptomatic or who has a dark discoloration on the sides or back of neck (acanthosis nigricans) should be tested. Ask your endocrinologist about other children.

There are numerous ongoing studies looking at the genetics of Type 1 diabetes. In most cases, the rate of development of diabetes in a child is 2 percent to 10 percent if a first-degree relative (sibling or parent) has the disorder. It is prudent to discuss with the endocrinologist what your other child's risk is, whether participation in a study is warranted, and if screening is recommended.

9. How often do I need to check back with you, and when do you wish to see my child again regarding this condition?

The pediatrician will work in conjunction with the pediatric endocrinologist, but in general, visits to the endocrinologist tend to be more frequent than visits to the pediatrician, whose role is general health maintenance and addressing nondiabetic medical concerns.

ELLEN S. SHER, MD
Endocrinology

DIAPER RASH

Definition: **Rash in the diaper area.**

Author's Comment: Try one of the over-the-counter preparations first, and keep your infant's diaper area as dry as possible. If the condition does not improve, contact your doctor because it may represent a yeast or some other type of infection that requires a prescription medication to get better.

1. What causes this condition, and how did my child contract it?

Diaper rash is very common and occurs because diaper area is covered and remains moist. Moist skin is more easily irritated, especially by repeated or prolonged contact with stool and urine. The result is red, inflamed, raw skin on the groin or buttocks. Diaper rash is most common in older infants who are sleeping through the night (due to less frequent diaper changes) or after a diarrhea illness.

2. Is it painful?

Diaper rash that is red and raw can be very tender. Painful skin should be cared for gently and simply with a minimum of creams or other products. Diaper wipes tend to sting when applied to irritated skin, so using a damp, soft washcloth to clean the skin would be better. Sitting the child in a tub of warm water is another way to keep the area clean, and this can be soothing, but even water may sting if the skin is inflamed enough. Since rubbing or touching the skin will hurt, diaper creams should be applied gently as a few thick globs without rubbing. The diaper cream will spread around on its own once the diaper is on.

3. How contagious is it?

Diaper rash is not contagious. Even diaper rash infected with yeast does not tend to be contagious. If it followed a diarrhea illness, however, the virus or bacteria that caused the diarrhea can be spread to others.

4. What is the treatment for this condition?

The most important thing is to keep the area clean and dry. Diapers should be changed more often, and the child should not be allowed to remain in a soiled diaper. The skin should also be protected from contact with moisture. This is best accomplished by liberal and frequent application of a thick zinc oxide or petrolatum-based diaper cream (the thicker the better) to serve as a protective barrier. Thick diaper creams do not need to be completely removed with every diaper change, as vigorous wiping will further irritate the skin—just wipe away the soiled top layer then apply more cream.

The goal is to treat the skin as gently as possible to allow it to heal. For those willing to assume the risk, allowing the child to "air out" and go without a diaper once in a while can help keep the area dry. If bright red bumps or pimple-like pus bumps are noted at the edges of the diaper rash, then there may be a superimposed yeast infection and use of an antiyeast cream two to three times a day will help.

5. How long will the rash persist once I begin the appropriate treatment?

Mild diaper rashes may improve within a few days, but more severe diaper rashes can persist for several weeks, particularly if diarrhea is present.

6. Will there be any scarring?

Scarring is uncommon, even after the worst looking diaper rashes, but it may take several weeks (up to a few months) for the skin redness to fade completely.

7. What can be done to prevent this condition from reoccurring?

Regular use of a thick diaper cream as a protective barrier and wipes that are fragrance and alcohol free is helpful. Also, children who are sleeping through the night should not be sent to bed with a bottle. To have a drier night, it is better to give the last bottle one to two hours before bedtime and change the diaper immediately before bed. Also, at the first sign of diarrhea, start changing the diapers more often— sitting too long in a soiled diaper one time is all it takes to start a diaper rash.

8. When do you wish to see my child again for this condition?

If the diaper rash does not show signs of improvement after a few days of basic treatment, if the skin bleeds, or if pus bumps are seen, then a follow-up visit may be needed.

K. ROBIN CARDER, MD
Dermatology

DIARRHEA

Definition: **Increase in frequency and fluidity of stools.**

Author's Comment: Follow the directions you receive from your doctor to make this condition improve. If the diarrhea persists, keep checking with the doctor because, although most diarrheas get better with simple dietary control, sometimes there can be an underlying cause that requires special treatment.

1. What is the cause of this condition, and how did my child contract it?

In a child who has no previous bouts of this problem, diarrhea is most often a result of an infection. Viral causes are perhaps the most common. It is contracted by a child from ingestion of the virus present on a contaminated material that was put in the mouth. The most talked-about is rotavirus. Other types of infection include bacterial (such as salmonella) and parasitic (such as giardia) infections.

2. Are there any other tests to be done, such as a stool culture or a parasite test to further define the cause?

If the diarrhea resolves after one to two days, doing stool tests is unnecessary. If it lasts for more than a few days, your doctor might order a bacterial culture, viral culture (or rotazyme), and/or ova and parasite tests on the stool.

3. How long will the diarrhea last?

Most diarrheal illnesses resulting from a viral infection last from a couple of days to about one week.

4. What is the treatment for this condition?

There is no treatment for viral diarrhea. Drinking plenty of fluids is important to avoid dehydration as a complication. Your doctor may recommend a lactose-free diet for a short period of time. A BRAT (banana, rice, apple sauce, toast) diet for a few days might also help, but it is important for children to continue eating during this illness to provide the nutrition needed to help fight the infection.

5. If I stop giving cow's milk to my child, when can I resume giving it?

About a week following complete recovery, most children are able to resume drinking milk and eating dairy products.

6. If I put my child on a limited diet, when will I know to progress the diet back to normal?

Once the diarrhea resolves, the child is usually able to resume a normal diet.

7. Are there any medicines to be given to slow down the diarrhea, and, if so, how long should they be used? What are the potential side effects of their usage?

Medicines to slow down the diarrhea are not safe to use in young children. These medications do not stop the excess fluid losses associated with the diarrhea. They only slow down the frequency of the bowel movements. The excess fluid is just stored inside the intestinal tract. As a result, parents are usually unaware that their child is losing a lot of fluids and are therefore unable to push more fluids by mouth.

8. What are the danger signs to look for if the diarrhea persists?

Dehydration is always a medical emergency. If your child cannot keep up with the fluid losses by drinking a lot, intravenous fluids through your local hospital emergency room may be necessary. These children usually have decreased urination, dry lips and mouth, and an inability to produce tears when they cry. Drowsiness and lethargy are often signs of severe dehydration.

9. When do I call you back if the diarrhea continues?

If the diarrhea persists for more than a week, if you see blood or mucous in the stool, if your child runs a fever, or if you have concerns about dehydration, make sure you inform your pediatrician.

10. Do you wish to see my child again regarding this condition?

If the child completely recovers from the diarrhea after a few days and has returned to normal activity and eating habits, a follow-up with your doctor is not necessary.

ERIC ARGAO, MD
Gastroenterology

DYSPLASIA (DEVELOPMENTAL) OF THE HIP

Definition: **Abnormal development of the hip.**

Author's Comment: This condition may not be present at birth and may be detected later on in infancy. This is one of the reasons you need to go back often for regular checkups during the first year of life. If detected early, this condition usually has a positive outcome.

1. What is the actual problem with the hip, and why did it occur?

The term "developmental dysplasia of the hip" (DDH) refers to several different anatomic abnormalities, from a slightly shallow socket in a hip that is properly located, to a poorly formed socket and dislocated hip. Many factors contribute to DDH. These include female gender, breech position, firstborn children, previous sibling with DDH, decreased amniotic fluid, and the presence of other musculoskeletal abnormalities.

2. What is the treatment, and should an orthopedist be consulted at this time?

The first goal of treatment in DDH is to obtain reduction (properly locate the hip joint) and maintain that reduction. Commonly, this can be done in the doctor's office by placing your child in a special soft harness (Pavlik harness) that maintains your child's hips in the proper position. If the hip joint cannot be placed or maintained in this manner, your child may need a surgical procedure to further study the abnormality or he or she may need to be placed in a body cast that holds the hip in proper position.

For cases of DDH in which this treatment is not successful, your child may require operative relocation and reconstruction of the hip joint when he or she is at least six months of age. Studies show that early diagnosis generally leads to a greater chance of successful treatment, so consultation with a pediatric orthopedist should occur soon after your pediatrician suspects your child may have DDH.

3. Is the condition totally correctable, or is it likely that there will be a residual problem?

With early diagnosis and successful treatment, DDH can be totally correctable. Occasionally, residual deformity requires surgery to improve the shape of the hip joint.

4. How long will it take for the prescribed treatment to correct this disorder?

If the Pavlik harness is successful at stabilizing an unstable hip, it is generally worn full time for six to twelve weeks, followed by six to twelve weeks of nap and nighttime wear. For children for which the harness treatment is not successful, the time to full correction depends on the extent of deformity and the surgical intervention necessary to achieve proper reduction and stabilization of the hip.

5. What type of restrictions will need to be imposed upon my child because of the disorder and the treatment?

While the Pavlik harness is worn, it is recommended to avoid tight-fitting clothes. During full-time harness use, sponge baths are necessary to bathe your child. You should also avoid the use of jumpers or walkers until your child is able to walk independently. The harness is generally worn during the first three to six months of life. If successful, this should not delay your child's walking, and there are no further restrictions. If only partial correction is achieved, further recommendations for treatment and subsequent activity restrictions would be individualized per child.

6. What kind of follow-up will be needed?

Following use of the Pavlik harness, your pediatric orthopedic surgeon will need to see your child weekly for the first two to three weeks to ensure proper hip position in the harness. Your child will then need to be seen at six-week intervals until the harness is discontinued. If the hip is developing normally at that point, your child will return every six months for an examination and X rays until approximately two to three years old.

RODERICK CAPELO, MD
Orthopedics

EAR INFECTION–MIDDLE EAR
(Otitis Media)

Definition: Infection of the middle ear.

Author's Comment: This condition frequently keeps parents up nights during a child's early years. It is definitely one of the common diseases that pediatricians see in their practice on a daily basis. In fact, I once contemplated changing our practice name to "Ear Infections Are Us." It is important that after you have finished the treatment regimen for your child's ear infection that you follow up with the doctor to make sure that the infection, as well as the fluid in the middle ear, has cleared to a satisfactory degree.

1. What causes this condition, and how did my child develop it?

Ear infections (otitis media) occur in the middle ear, the space behind the eardrum (tympanic membrane). The middle ear is connected to the back of the nasal cavity (nasopharynx) by a tube called the eustachian tube. Ear infections occur because of dysfunction in the eustachian tube.

The eustachian tube is the body's natural way to ventilate the middle ear, to allow fluid to drain when the ear is infected, and to allow air to enter the ear and keep it healthy. A child's eustachian tube does not function as well as an adult's for a variety of reasons. In young children the eustachian tube has a flat (more horizontal) angle in relationship to the base of the skull. During the first few years of life the angle changes rapidly and is believed to decrease the risk of developing ear infections. Other differences in the eustachian tube of children compared to adults include softer tube cartilage and less developed muscles that open the tube. The tube typically matures toward the adult levels of function by age six to eight years.

In addition to problems with the eustachian tube, young children have immature immune systems and may be exposed to other sick children. The exposure to other sick children is increased in the daycare or school setting. Upper respiratory infections may cause swelling around the opening or in the wall of the eustachian tube preventing ventilation of the middle ear.

Another consideration is the adenoid. The adenoid is a pad of soft tissue (much like the tonsils) that is positioned in the back of the nasal cavity (the nasopharynx) that may obstruct the opening of the eustachian tube or provide bacterial contamination of one end of the eustachian tube.

The eustachian tube is controlled by muscles in the soft palate. Children with a cleft palate typically have abnormal eustachian tube function and a higher risk for developing ear infections.

2. What medicines are needed to combat this infection?

Not all ear infections require antibiotics for treatment. Purulent fluid (pus) is what is seen when a child has the typical findings of fever, pain, pulling at the ears, or increased irritability. Children with this type of ear infection should always be treated with antibiotics. Antibiotics can be administered orally or with an intramuscular injection.

Serous fluid (thin clear yellow fluid) and mucoid fluid (very thick glue-like fluid) often lack many of the symptoms of purulent fluid. Often the primary symptom of children with this type of fluid is hearing loss related to the presence of the fluid. This type of fluid may resolve without antibiotics, depending upon the entire clinical picture.

There are a number of other medications (nasal steroid sprays, oral steroids, antihistamines, and decongestants) that are occasionally used in children with middle ear fluid. These are not generally recommended since a clear benefit has not been shown, and they may have undesirable side effects. There are certain patients, such as those with allergies, who may benefit from some of these medications.

3. What medicines can I give my child to relieve the pain?

The pain of an ear infection can usually be treated with acetaminophen or ibuprofen. These medications will also help to reduce the fever that may be associated with your child's ear infection. Your physician may prescribe ear drops for pain or, at times, an oral narcotic pain reliever when the pain is intense.

4. Are there any side effects associated with the medicines used in the treatment of this condition?

Any therapy has potential side effects. Treatment with antibiotics has the potential for the development of diarrhea, nausea, vomiting, rash, or allergic reaction. Treatment with antihistamines or steroid nose sprays may lead to nasal dryness and even nose bleeds. The risk of surgeries should be discussed with your surgeon.

5. After treatment has started, when should I see improvement?

Improvement in fevers and irritability is usually seen within twenty-four to forty-eight hours after starting antibiotic therapy. Hearing loss related to the fluid in the middle ear may take weeks or months to improve.

6. What can be done to prevent this condition from reoccurring?

Avoiding environments that increase your child's risk of developing an upper respiratory infection (daycare or interactions with ill children) will decrease his or her risk of developing an ear infection. Avoiding secondhand smoke exposure (which includes the smell of smoke on a caregiver's clothes) will also decrease his or her risk of developing an ear infection.

There are some vaccines that may be effective in certain cases; these should be discussed with your pediatrician.

Although a variety of allergies can contribute to swelling in the lining of the nose and in the drainage pathway of the ear (the eustachian tube), allergies will usually cause other symptoms in addition to ear infections. It is uncommon to have ear infections as the only sign/symptom of an allergy. Treating allergies may decrease your child's risk of developing ear infections.

In certain chronic situations consultation with an ear, nose, and throat (ENT) specialist to discuss ventilation tubes for the ears may be recommended.

7. In the case of recurrent ear infections, should we consider ventilation tubes, and when should we see an ENT specialist?

Children with persistent ear fluid or multiple recurrent ear infections may be offered surgery. This is usually a last resort after it has become clear that nonsurgical treatment is not helping, or that the risks of medical treatment (such as reactions to antibiotics) are too high. If the middle ear fluid has persisted for two to three months, it is less likely that the fluid will resolve on its own. Middle ear fluid is often associated with hearing loss. Children with persistent middle ear fluid (two to three months) and hearing loss may need surgery (ventilation tubes).

A child that has had more than five or six ear infections in a year, and the medical treatment described above has not been successful in controlling the problem, the child may need surgery (ventilation tubes). The surgery done for chronic or recurrent ear infections is known as pressure equalizing tube placement. The tubes are for ventilation of the middle ear.

8. How can one be sure that there is no permanent hearing loss associated with this condition?

Permanent hearing loss from recurrent or chronic ear infections is very uncommon. The hearing loss associated with ear infections is typically related to the fluid in the middle ear limiting the movement of sound into the inner ear. When the middle ear fluid resolves, the hearing typically returns to normal.

Typically when your child is evaluated by an ENT specialist, a hearing test is completed as part of the initial evaluation and is repeated when the middle ear fluid has resolved.

9. When do you wish to see my child again regarding this condition?

The ear should be reassessed in four to six weeks unless symptoms such as fever or increased irritability develop. When a middle ear is treated with antibiotics, the middle ear is typically reevaluated in two to three weeks to assess response to the antibiotic used. If fevers or increased irritability persist for more than forty-eight hours after antibiotic therapy is started, you should contact your physician. In some cases the bacteria may be resistant to the antibiotic chosen for therapy.

PAUL W. BAUER, MD
Otolaryngology

EAR INFECTION–OUTER EAR
(Otitis Externa)

Definition: Inflammation of the outer canal of the ear.

Author's Comment: This is the so-called swimmer's ear type infection. A lot of these external ear infections do not occur from swimming but are caused when contaminated water from any source accumulates in the external ear resulting in inflammation and infection. Once your child has had swimmer's ear, it is advisable in most situations to use preventative drops whenever the child goes swimming in the future.

1. What is the cause of this condition, and how did my child contract it?

Otitis externa (OE) is an inflammation of the external ear canal, usually caused by a bacterial infection. It can also be caused by a yeast or fungal infection, or by general skin conditions such as eczema. OE differs from acute otitis media (AOM), the more common type of childhood ear infection, in that OE involves the ear canal, whereas AOM refers to an infection behind the eardrum (in the middle ear).

Also, with OE there may be tenderness of the external ear, ear drainage, and swelling of the ear canal.

OE results from contamination of the ear canal with bacteria, usually water borne (hence the term "swimmer's ear"). Predisposing medical factors may include excessive or insufficient cerumen (ear wax), dermatitis (skin conditions), trauma, foreign bodies, and medical conditions such as diabetes. Swimming in oceans and lakes does not necessarily predispose to OE (so long as the water is clean). Hot, sunny weather can decompose chlorine in pools more quickly, resulting in pool water becoming contaminated more easily.

2. What is the treatment for this condition, and how long should it be continued?

Initial treatment for OE is usually topical in the form of eardrops. Eardrops for treatment of OE contain antibiotics and also may contain a steroid or other medications to reduce inflammation. The pH of the medication is also important, as an acidic drop (low pH) will also help kill bacteria. If significant ear canal inflammation is present, a wick may be placed to help deliver the medication to the ear canal. Failure of topical therapy or infection that has spread to the external ear may require an oral antibiotic. Occasionally, debris in the ear canal may require cleaning of the ear canal as part of treatment.

3. What are the potential side effects from the treatment?

The most common side effect of treatment is treatment failure, when symptoms fail to subside with twenty-four to forty-eight hours of treatment. If this occurs, further treatments may be necessary, such as cleaning of the ear canal or oral antibiotic therapy. Other side effects may include ear pain with administration of the eardrops. This typically results from the acidity of the drops. Causes of ear pain may be the presence of an ear tube or an unrecognized perforation of the eardrum.

Allergy to certain antibiotics is also a common side effect. Typical reactions are redness and irritation of the skin, often caused by medications such as Neomycin. Newer antibiotics, such as Cipro or Floxin, are less likely to result in an allergic reaction. Prolonged use of antibiotic eardrops may result in yeast or fungal infection, which may require prolonged treatment.

4. How long will it take for the ear pain to subside?

With adequate treatment, pain should subside within twenty-four to forty-eight hours. It is important that adequate pain relief be given. In many cases ibuprofen (Motrin or Advil) may be adequate; however, narcotic pain medication can be required because of the severity of the pain. As mentioned previously, failure for the pain to subside with one to two days of treatment may signal that additional treatment is required.

5. When can my child resume putting his or her head under water?

While acute symptoms such as pain, tenderness, pronounced swelling, or ear drainage are present, swimming is probably not advisable. Once these acute symptoms have improved, water exposure most likely will not interfere with treatment so long as medication is applied after swimming. Prolonged exposure to water, however, is probably not advisable until full recovery.

6. What can be done to prevent this condition from recurring?

An acidified alcohol eardrop such as Swim Ear can be used, though in general no preventative treatment is necessary. Prior to using an alcohol eardrop, it is important to be sure that a perforation or an ear tube is not present in the eardrum, as drainage of alcohol behind the eardrum will result in significant pain.

7. When do you wish to see my child again regarding this condition?

If symptoms resolve with initial treatment, follow-up is generally not necessary. Failure for symptoms to improve within one to two days should trigger a visit to the physician for additional treatment. If a wick is placed, or if cleaning of the ear canal is required, a one-week follow-up is usually needed. If a yeast or fungal infection is present, several visits may be required for cleaning of the ear canal until the infection resolves.

MICHAEL BIAVATI, MD
Otolaryngology

EAR WAX IMPACTION
(Cerumen Impaction)

Definition: Ear wax lodged in and blocking the ear canal.

Author's Comment: This is relatively common and, at times, is so severe that it can impair hearing and indirectly lead to external ear infections. It seems like every doctor has a different approach to dealing with this problem and removing the wax.

1. What causes this condition?

Earwax impaction is a common condition that can occur at any age. The most common cause is improper cleaning with a cotton swab or frequent ear examinations. Another common cause is a genetic predisposition to earwax that is either too dry or too sticky. Foreign bodies, including ear tubes (grommets) that have fallen into the ear canal can lead to abnormal wax buildup. Children who wear hearing aids may also be prone to earwax impaction due to constant presence of the earmold.

2. What can be done to make it better?

Treatment of ear wax impaction often requires removal of the excess wax, either with an ear curette (an instrument with a loop on the end) or suction. In some cases where the impaction does not extend to the eardrum, over-the-counter medications such as Debrox can be used. In general, flushing (irrigation) of the ear canal is not recommended as this may be painful and can lead to an infection of the ear canal (swimmer's ear).

3. Does the condition impair my child's hearing?

Earwax impaction does not cause long-term hearing loss. Blockage of the ear canal with cerumen can lead to significant hearing loss. This would be similar to wearing earplugs on an ongoing basis.

4. What danger is created by leaving the wax alone, as is?

Left untreated, impacted earwax can lead to an infection of the ear canal. More commonly, the presence of excessive earwax can make examination of the ear difficult. As discussed previously, blockage of the ear canal with wax may cause hearing loss.

5. What is "candling," and is it applicable for this disorder?

Ear candling is a homeopathic treatment for excessive earwax and other general ear conditions. Candling is done by placing a cone of beeswax at the ear canal and lighting the open end. The resultant airflow created by the flame is intended to draw wax and other illnesses from the ear. No benefit has ever been shown by candling; in fact, injury may result from melted wax burning the skin of the external ear.

6. Are there any preventive measures that can be taken to keep this condition from reoccurring?

The ear canal is designed to be self-cleaning, and earwax assists in this function. Left alone, cerumen normally works its way out of the canal taking along dirt and debris accumulated in the canal. Manipulation of the earwax, such as with cleaning with cotton swabs or frequent ear examinations, can interrupt this normal flow. For children with frequent buildup of earwax, medications such Debrox can help prevent buildup. If removal of the earwax by your physician is required, periodic visits for cleaning may be beneficial.

7. What kind of follow-up is needed in the future?

Follow-up for children with recurrent significant buildup of earwax typically is every four to six months. If symptoms (such as hearing loss) recur, sooner follow-up is indicated.

MICHAEL BIAVATI, MD
Otolaryngology

EATING DISORDERS
(e.g., Bulimia, Anorexia)

Definition: Pathologic disturbance of the eating pattern.

Author's Comment: It seems that these types of disorders are becoming more and more prevalent, especially in our teenage population. It is probably a consequence of multiple factors, including family tendencies, peer pressures, school stress, and our fast-paced society. A multipronged approach is needed for treatment.

1. What causes children to experience this kind of disorder?

There are many reasons that factor into the development of an eating disorder. We tend to live in a society in which food is prevalent and, at the same time, being considered attractive is linked to being fit. Western societies suffer the most from development of eating disorders that are linked to unrealistic social expectations. The U.S. and Canada have among the highest rates of eating disorders in the world. Other factors that are thought to be significant causes are the prevalence of anxiety and depressive disorder. Obsessive-compulsive disorder (OCD) especially can be linked with eating disorders, and many clinicians believe that eating disorders are a subtype of OCD.

2. What are some of the issues that need to be discussed and explored to further define the problem area?

Within the family system, parents must strongly take a look at the messages, either verbal or nonverbal, that they are sending to their children. Eating as a means of comforting oneself is a very common coping strategy that we have all used at one time or another. Parents will often seek to focus on a child's appetite and weight to deal with their own anxiety or feelings of "being out of control" with other aspects of their life. These negative messages or negative parent coping strategies can be linked to some of the child's development of self-perceptions that become askew and inaccurate.

3. How does one differentiate whether this is a phase as opposed to a more serious long-term disorder?

Certainly adolescents can go through "phases" where they focus on losing weight and tend to accomplish this through dieting or restricting. These seem to be self-contained episodes. They may often be linked to making sports teams or a cheerleading squad. However, if this restricted behavior pattern extends beyond a few weeks or begins to lead to rapid weight loss or undernourishment one must consider that a more serious eating disorder is developing. Often children develop a very distorted body image that can lead to a more significant binge/purge pattern, excessive exercise, or the use of dieting products. Laxatives and diuretics are often used and would again represent a significant increase in escalation of the problem.

4. Can depression be an underlying issue?

Depression is clearly an underlying issue in most eating disorders. Self-image, poor body image, and low self-esteem are very frequently linked with eating disorders.

5. What can I do to make it better and to help my child overcome this disorder?

Sending positive and encouraging messages is the best intervention, along with close monitoring of the situation. Parents have had their greatest success when they can align themselves with their child and together develop healthy nutritional plans and exercise plans in which the whole family can become involved in which the child is not meant to feel like a "scapegoat."

6. Is it necessary to consult a nutritionist?

A nutritionist may be consulted to offer guidance in what are appropriate dietary guidelines for a preadolescent or adolescent and most certainly would be needed if weight loss has become a trend that is difficult to stop.

7. Is the timing right to consult a psychologist or psychiatrist?

Often a psychologist can be greatly beneficial to help a child identify some of the root causes of his or her eating disorder. Self-esteem, body image, peer pressure, and family conflicts can often be identified as being at the root of a budding eating disorder. A psychologist would also be able to identify whether a bigger clinical picture may be developing of a mood or an anxiety disorder that might require further medication intervention and referral to a psychiatrist.

8. Is there any medication that can be used to help treat this condition?

Most of the medications that are considered in the treatment of eating disorders often tend to focus on the underlying depressive or anxiety features. Medication intervention can be equally beneficial to those mood or anxiety disorders and the eating disorder.

9. Are there any side effects from the medicine?

All medications can have a side-effect profile, and the decision to medicate is not made lightly. A psychiatrist can help navigate you through a variety of those choices. This, again, is based on appropriateness of that intervention and strongly considering therapeutic benefits versus the potential side effects.

10. How often does my child need to be weighed?

Monitoring a child's weight may need to occur quite often if the weight loss is a specific concern. However, the process of monitoring a child's weight can often play into the pathology of the disorder and usually needs to be done in the office of a nutritionist or pediatrician. Many parents are instructed to remove scales from the homes and to put behavior intervention in place so that a specific number does not end up being a focus for their child.

11. When do you wish to see my child again for this disorder?

As with a mood or anxiety disorder, children with an eating disorder must be monitored closely. Untreated eating disorders tend to have a high rate of injury and can even, at worse case scenario, have a mortality factor associated with them. Intervention in eating disorders should be early and often.

DANTE BURGOS, MD
Psychiatry

ECZEMA

Definition: An inflammatory, red, itchy, scaly skin condition with, at times, watery discharge and the development of crusts or scabs.

Author's Comment: This is a common skin condition in youngsters that many (but not all) children eventually outgrow. In the meantime, keep using the lubricants, special skin cleansers, and creams that your doctor prescribes.

1. What causes this condition to occur in my child? Is it hereditary?

The cause of eczema is not clear. There are many factors involved rather than one isolated cause. In many cases, the tendency to develop eczema is inherited, and family members of affected children often have eczema, dry or sensitive skin, hay fever allergies, or asthma themselves.

In general, eczema is a type of dry, sensitive skin that children are born with, although the overt signs of eczema may not appear until later infancy or childhood. Our skin serves as a protective outer cover keeping moisture in and keeping irritating things out. The skin barrier in children with eczema is defective; moisture leaks out, irritating things enter, and the skin becomes red, dry, and itchy. If the skin remains irritated, a vicious cycle of itching and scratching begins, and the skin barrier worsens, leading to more inflammation.

2. What are the different ways of treating this condition, and what medicines can be used?

There are three steps to treating eczema: (1) repair the skin barrier with gentle skin care and moisturizers, (2) treat the inflammation, and (3) treat any secondary skin infections. It is very important to understand that eczema is a chronic (long-term) condition that comes and goes. Although eczema tends to improve with age, we have no quick-fix cure. Treatment is aimed at first getting the eczema under control, then maintaining that improvement and treating temporary flare-ups.

The most important step is to repair the skin barrier with moisturizers. Soaking in a comfortably warm (but not hot) bath for twenty minutes followed by liberally applying a moisturizer helps to add moisture back to the skin. Because perfume and fragrances can be irritating to sensitive skin, fragrance-free moisturizers are recommended. If your child's skin is very dry, then a heavier cream or ointment (petroleum jelly-like) moisturizer would be preferred over a thin lotion.

Moisturizers should be used every day—even when there are no active eczema lesions—as a preventative measure to maintain a healthy skin barrier. Because keeping the skin hydrated is so crucial to the treatment of eczema, this has been a topic of much recent research. As a result, several new moisturizers are now available that are specifically designed to correct and repair the abnormal skin barrier of children with eczema.

For skin inflammation (red, scaly, itchy spots) that does not improve with moisturizers alone, topical anti-inflammatory creams containing either cortisone (steroid) or certain nonsteroid (tacrolimus or pimecrolimus) medications are used. These medications help to decrease the redness, itching, and inflammation of the skin. They should be applied as a thin layer one to two times a day to the active (red, scaly) eczema lesions only; they should not be applied to normal (smooth feeling) skin. The medication should be used consistently until the skin feels normal (smooth) again. Once improvement is achieved, the creams are used on an as-needed basis to treat lesions as they return. Because oral steroids and steroid injections have a greater potential for side effects and provide only temporary benefit but no continued improvement or maintenance benefit, they are not ideal eczema treatments. Oral antihistamines can be very helpful for control of itching, particularly at night when children tend to scratch the most.

Lastly, children with eczema are more prone to develop secondary bacterial or viral skin infections. They tend to have many areas of open skin due to scratching that provide a site of entry for bacteria. Signs of infection include boils (deep, tender knots in the skin), pus bumps, honey-colored crusting, or blisters. If any of these signs are noted, then follow-up with your doctor is recommended, and treatment with an appropriate antibiotic or antiviral medication may be needed. If your child has fever of 100.5 degrees or more along with signs of a skin infection, then hospitalization for intravenous therapy may be required.

3. How long will it take for this condition to show improvement?

The rate of improvement depends on the thickness and duration of the skin lesions. Newer, thin, pink, scaly spots will improve in a few days to a week. Older, thick, or leathery eczema lesions (such as those on the hands, feet, elbows, and knees) may require three to four weeks of daily treatment to clear up. If the skin does not respond to treatment as expected, either the anti-inflammatory cream is not strong enough, the skin is infected, or there is another aggravating factor such as a food allergy or nighttime scratching that may need to be addressed.

4. What are factors that may worsen or aggravate eczema?

There are many factors that aggravate (but are not the cause of) eczema. Cold, dry weather or hot, humid weather can make eczema worse. As a general rule, heat and sweating make the skin itch more, so it is important to keep your child's room cool and not over bundle him or her with heavy clothes or blankets. If you live in a hot climate, then keeping your child in a cool, air-conditioned environment (i.e., keeping him or her indoors during recess or physical education class) on very hot days may help. Wool clothing is prickly and very irritating to children with eczema; soft cotton clothes are best.

Synthetic fabrics like polyester do not breathe and may aggravate eczema. Stress and emotions are common triggers of flare-ups. Some laundry detergents that contain fragrances or dyes can irritate the skin; using a fragrance- and dye-free detergent or running your clothes through a second rinse cycle can help. Also, certain creams or lotions may irritate the skin in children with eczema. In general, ointments contain fewer additives than creams and lotions, so they tend to be less irritating. If your child's medication or moisturizer seems to sting or burn when you put it on, then changing to an ointment form may help.

Lastly, skin infections cause eczema to worsen and should be looked for if the cause of the flare-up is not clear. That being said, sometimes eczema worsens for no good reason even if you are doing everything right, so do your best and control the things that you can, but do not take the flare-ups personally.

5. How often should my child bathe?

This has been a source of debate for a long time. In general, you should not bathe your child more than once a day, and you should apply the medicated creams and moisturizers immediately afterward. Nevertheless, a recent study seems to indicate that every other day bathing may be best.

6. How should I use the moisturizers and medicines?

In general, the medicated creams should be applied to the individual eczema lesions first. Then the moisturizer should be applied to the entire body. If no active eczema lesions are present, only the moisturizer should be used. Never use your prescription anti-inflammatory cream as a moisturizer.

7. If used, are there any potential side effects from these medicines?

In the community, there is a lot of fear, rumor, and misinformation surrounding topical steroids. It must be remembered that these medications come in a wide variety of strengths, the mildest being hydrocortisone. When anti-inflammatory creams of an appropriate strength are used correctly, they are quite safe, and side effects are rare. Using potent topical steroids on areas of fragile skin, such as the face, neck, underarms, or groin, would not be appropriate and could potentially cause thinning of the skin (stretch marks) over time. Nevertheless, even the most potent topical steroids have their place and would be appropriate for use on thick, long-standing eczema lesions on less delicate skin sites, such as the palms and soles.

Steroids do have the potential to cause weight gain, mood changes, high blood pressure, eye changes, or slowed growth (height), but these side effects are rare with topical steroids and typically only occur with repeated use of oral or injected steroids. Because steroid creams are applied to the skin only and are not used internally, very little of the medication is absorbed, and the risk of internal side effects from intermittent topical use is low. The medications should be used appropriately and as directed by your physician.

Problems are more likely to occur if you take matters into your own hands and use your child's stronger body medication on a delicate area like the face, for example. If the directions say twice daily, do not apply the cream three or four times a day. As a general rule, you should not apply the medication to areas of normal (unaffected) skin—in other words, it is not good to use your medicated cream as a moisturizer for full body use, unless your child has eczema lesions that cover every inch of his or her body.

Lastly, because all of the anti-inflammatory medications decrease inflammation by suppressing the immune system to some degree, some of these medications may increase the likelihood of getting a skin infection. That being said, skin infections are more likely to occur if the eczema is not treated, so do not be afraid to use your medications. Remember, side effects are uncommon when you follow your doctor's instructions and use the medications appropriately.

8. Are there any allergic factors involved? If so, do we need to test for them?

A subset of children with eczema may have some form of allergies. They may have hay fever allergies, which cause sneezing and watery eyes after exposure to dust, plant pollens, mold, or animal dander. Others may have allergies to certain foods, such as milk, soy, peanut, egg, and wheat. Only about 10 percent to 20 percent of children with moderate to severe eczema will have food allergies.

It is very important to understand that the food allergies do not cause the eczema. Many people cling to the hope that if they can identify and eliminate the one magic food that is causing the problem, then their child will be cured of eczema forever. This is rarely the case. The eczema may get a little better after the food your child is allergic to is eliminated from the diet, but the eczema will still be there, and the skin will continue to need treatment.

Testing for food allergies can be done easily with a blood test, but these blood tests are not very reliable under the age of one year. Allergy testing would be recommended for children with moderate-to-severe eczema that does not clear up as expected with standard treatment. Testing would also be a good idea if your child gets hives, stomach upset, or eczema flare-ups every time that he or she eats a particular food. Randomly taking food out of your child's diet without a doctor's supervision or proper testing is not recommended.

9. Are there any dietary modifications needed?

For most children with eczema, no change in diet is needed. If your child has a known food allergy, then that food should be avoided. Avoidance can be tricky since some foods, such as peanuts, can be present in small amounts and not obvious, so a consultation with an allergist may help you understand what foods your child can and cannot eat. Since milk and soy formulas are the main source of protein for growing babies, these foods should not be eliminated from your child's diet without a doctor's supervision, and a suitable milk substitute would need to be started. An example of a poor milk substitute would be rice milk, which does not contain enough protein for a growing child.

As your child gets older, some food allergies fade away, so repeating allergy testing around three years of age may be helpful. If the food allergy has resolved, then that food can gradually be added back to your child's diet.

10. Will the condition cause any permanent scarring?

As bad as the eczema may look at times, scarring is rare. The skin may be discolored (red, light, or dark) for several months, but this fades over time and is not permanent. When scarring does occur, it is usually the result of picking or vigorous scratching of the skin by fingernails, not from the eczema itself.

11. What symptoms would warrant seeing an allergist or a dermatologist?

If your child has more severe eczema that fails to clear up (at least for a little while) following basic treatment with moisturizers and a low-to-medium potency anti-inflammatory cream, then it may be time to get additional help. Consultation with a dermatologist is useful to optimize the treatment plan or to determine if there are additional problems, such as a skin infection, that are preventing the skin from clearing up. A visit with an allergist may be helpful to determine if food allergies are present or to manage hay fever allergies or asthma, conditions that can accompany eczema.

12. When do I call you back if I do not feel the condition is improving adequately?

With appropriate treatment, even the most stubborn skin lesions should improve within three to four weeks. If the skin lesions do not improve or clear up within a few weeks, then you should let your doctor know. If the eczema lesions clear up and then come back once you stop using the medicine, this is normal and expected. It does not mean that your treatment failed. Eczema will come and go no matter what treatment is used, since we have no cure to make the skin lesions stay gone forever. What we can do is get the skin lesions to clear up and then keep them under control with periodic maintenance treatment and daily dry skin care.

13. When do you wish to see my child again for this condition?

If your child has signs of a skin infection (blisters, pus bumps, crusting, oozing, fever), then you need to see your doctor. Also, if your child is no longer responding to the same treatment that used to work well, then your child may need to return for follow-up so that the treatment plan can be adjusted. If the eczema affects your child's school performance or if your child seems depressed because of his or her skin condition, you should let your doctor know.

K. ROBIN CARDER, MD
Dermatology

EYE INFECTION
(Conjunctivitis)

Definition: Inflammation of the outer lining of the eye.

Author's Comment: This is the condition that is commonly called "pink eye." In the contagious types, usually your child only has to be isolated for a day or two once appropriate therapy begins.

1. What causes this condition, and how did my child contract it?

There are many causes of conjunctivitis (or pink eye). The most common are allergic, viral, and bacterial. Allergic conjunctivitis is very common and involves both eyes. It is not contagious and is typically related to seasonal allergies. Viral and bacterial conjunctivitis usually begin as an infection of one eye and may be contagious for several days. These types of "pink eye" may be passed by hand-to-hand contact or the sharing of cups, towels, and so on.

2. Will this condition cause any permanent damage to the eyes?

If treated properly, these conditions rarely cause permanent damage to the eyes.

3. How is it treated and for how long?

Allergic conjunctivitis is typically treated with antihistamine drops as needed. For severe forms, steroid drops may be necessary. Bacterial conjunctivitis is almost always treated with antibiotic drops, usually for five to seven days. Viral conjunctivitis does not respond to anti-bacterial drops, but they may be used to prevent a secondary infection. These conditions also may improve with cold compresses and artificial tears to ease the discomfort.

4. If medicines are used, are there any potential side effects that can occur?

As with any medicine, there are side effects that may occur, particularly if they are used improperly. Antibiotic drops should be used as prescribed. Overuse may result in injury to the surface of the eye, and improper use may result in exacerbation of the infection. Steroid drops, which may be used for allergic conjunctivitis, are particularly dangerous if improperly used.

5. How long does it take to get over this condition?

The duration of symptoms may last several days or months depending on the cause. Viral and bacterial conjunctivitis typically resolve within seven to ten days if properly treated. Allergic conjunctivitis is typically seasonal and may last for weeks or months if not treated.

6. Is this condition contagious and, if so, for how long?

Viral conjunctivitis is typically contagious for the first four to seven days. Bacterial conjunctivitis may be contagious for one to three days after treatment is instituted, depending on the type of infection and the medicine used. Allergic conjunctivitis is not contagious. Contact your doctor for specific information regarding the contagious nature of any particular episode.

7. When should we call you back if we do not think the medicine is working?

You should contact your doctor immediately if the symptoms are worsening despite treatment. You should also contact your doctor if symptoms are not improving after several days of treatment.

8. When do you wish to see my child again for this condition?

If the symptoms resolve with proper treatment, it is not necessary to see your doctor again. If the symptoms recur, however, you should contact your doctor.

DAVID STAGER, JR, MD
Ophthalmology

EYELID GLAND SWELLING
(Chalazion)

Definition: **An inflammatory eyelid mass.**

Author's Comment: Most of these eyelid swellings get better on their own over a period of time, but sometimes this just does not happen. Keep in touch with your child's doctor regarding treatment. Generally, this condition does not cause any harm.

1. What causes this condition, and how did my child contract it?

An inflammatory eyelid mass (chalazion) is caused by a blockage of an oil gland of the eyelid. It is not contagious and does not result from an infection. A blockage of the oil gland results in an inflammatory reaction that causes the swelling.

2. How painful does it get?

A chalazion may be mildly tender in the early stages, but it is typically not painful.

3. Can it damage the eye or eyelid?

Chalazia rarely cause damage to the eye or eyelid.

4. What other problems or dangers does it pose?

The major problem with a chalazion is that it may be a cosmetic concern. It is also prone to recurrence.

5. What is the treatment, and do antibodies help?

Warm compresses are the best initial treatment. Antibiotics do not help, since this is not a result of an infection. For severe chronic chalazia, steroid injections, or surgical removal may be used.

6. If medicines are prescribed, what are their potential side effects, and how long should they be taken?

Medicines are rarely prescribed for this condition. Your doctor may prescribe an antibiotic drop or ointment if there is concern over a secondary infection. These medicines should be taken as prescribed. Side effects may include allergic reaction to the antibiotic as well as irritation of the eye or skin.

7. How long does it take for this condition to resolve?

Chalazia typically improve over several weeks with warm compresses. In a minority of patients, chalazia may be chronic and require surgical removal.

8. Will surgery ever be needed?

Surgery is an option for chronic, unsightly chalazia.

9. Do we need to consult an ophthalmologist?

Ophthalmologists are frequently consulted for severe, chronic, or recurrent chalazia. You should consult with your doctor if the chalazion is worsening or fails to improve after one month.

10. When do you wish to see my child again for this condition?

Your doctor should be contacted again if the eyelid swelling is getting bigger or more painful, or does not improve over a period of six to eight weeks.

DAVID STAGER, JR, MD
Ophthalmology

EYE MUSCLE IMBALANCE
(Strabismus)

Definition: Tight or weak eye muscles (eye muscle imbalance), causing a misalignment of the eyes (strabismus).

Author's Comment: You need to see a pediatric ophthalmologist for this condition. The nice thing to know is that it is usually correctable.

1. What is the cause of this condition, and how did it occur in my child?

Strabismus (misalignment of the eyes) may be present at birth or develop over time. The causes are many, but an eye muscle imbalance (tight or weak eye muscles) or significant farsightedness (poor focus of the eye) are the most common causes. Strabismus may also be associated with other systemic medical problems.

2. Will it correct itself, or will surgery be required?

Many newborns will show evidence of strabismus. The vast majority will straighten in the first few months of life. Patients who continue to have misalignment of the eyes beyond four to six months, or who develop strabismus later, almost always require treatment.

3. Is there any other treatment for this condition other than surgery?

Glasses are frequently used to treat strabismus. Patching, eye drops, and, in a few cases, eye exercises may also be effective in treating strabismus.

4. Does it affect the vision? If so, will the vision return to normal with treatment?

Strabismus does affect the vision by disrupting "fusion" or the use of the eyes together. It may also cause decreased vision, which is referred to as amblyopia or "lazy eye." Treatment is aimed at restoring normal vision and is often successful if the problem is treated promptly.

5. When do we need to see an ophthalmologist, and are there ones that specialize in this condition?

As soon as you or your doctor feel there is a problem, you should consult with an ophthalmologist. Pediatric ophthalmologists are specifically trained to treat strabismus.

6. When do you wish to see my child again for this disorder?

Your doctor may want to see your child every two to three months if the strabismus is suspected or intermittent. If it progresses, your child should see an eye doctor.

DAVID STAGER, JR, MD
Ophthalmology

FAILURE TO THRIVE

Definition: Not gaining weight or growing
               adequately.

Author's Comment: This is a complicated condition to sort out. There can be some underlying medical disorder going on, but at times, no such cause is definable. In addition to your child's doctor, other specialists and caretakers frequently need to be involved. It is important that your child be followed closely until the condition is resolved.

1. What is the cause of this condition, and how did my child contract it?

The causes of failure to thrive (FTT) are best broken down into two categories: medical or psychosocial. The medical causes can be from decreased caloric intake, inadequate digestion of nutrients, and increased caloric requirements. Some of the diseases are congenital such as cystic fibrosis, congenital heart disease, and metabolic defects. A child or infant may develop FTT over time from diseases such as inflammatory bowel disease, celiac disease (gluten intolerance), postviral inflammation of the intestines, and endocrine disorders (growth hormone or thyroid deficiency).

Psychosocial causes include caloric deprivation associated with poverty, parental choices, cultural or religious norms; behavioral issues that a child might have developed toward feeding (aversion); or child neglect.

2. What diagnostic tests are necessary to further define what is going on?

A good history, dietary evaluation, and physical examination, including weight and height measurements, are very important. The stool may be tested for malabsorption of fat and sugars and to exclude infections such as parasites. Blood work includes a complete blood count, serum electrolytes, liver and kidney function tests, total protein measurements and albumin testing. If celiac disease is considered, a celiac panel (specific blood testes) might be ordered.

3. What is the proposed treatment?

The treatment depends upon the cause of the FTT. In most cases, treating the disease takes care of the FTT, but nutritional rehabilitation is an integral part of therapy. An example would be a gluten-free diet in a patient with celiac disease. Children with inadequate caloric intake require high-calorie food supplementation. Psychosocial issues, including but not limited to child neglect, are sometimes best addressed with admittance to the hospital.

4. What are the potential problems that could result from this condition, and what is the long-term outlook for my child?

It is important to aggressively treat the FTT to prevent malnutrition and its complications, such as increased risk of infections, developmental delay, and vitamin deficiencies. The long-term outlook depends upon the cause of the FTT.

5. Do we need to consult with any specialists regarding this condition?

A specialist is required when there is involvement of a particular organ system. A pediatric gastroenterologist sees patients with inflammatory bowel disease, celiac disease, and severe gastroesophageal acid reflux. A pulmonologist manages patients with cystic fibrosis and chronic lung disease. A nephrologist (kidney specialist) takes care of patients with chronic renal failure or cystic kidney disease. If there are behavioral issues with feeding, a feeding therapist may have to be involved.

6. Does the diet need to be modified?

Nutritional rehabilitation is very important in the treatment of FTT. The dietary modification is dependent upon the disease. If there is any intolerance to carbohydrates, fat, or protein, the offending agent should be eliminated or modified. Any underlying disease will have to be treated. At the same time, extra calories for catch-up growth will have to be provided.

7. What kind of follow-up is needed?

Weekly follow-up for infants, and every two weeks in older children should focus on weight measurement and evaluation for any improvement in symptoms. Once weight gain is noted and symptoms have improved, follow-up can be done every few months until resolution of the FTT. Usually, the infant or child requires additional follow-up by the subspecialist consulted for the particular organ system that is involved.

ANNETTE WHITNEY, MD
Gastroenterology

FAINTING
(Syncope)

Definition: An episode characterized by a temporary loss of consciousness.

Author's Comment: This may not be as prevalent a condition today as it was during your grandmother's time. Nonetheless, it still does happen and poses a danger for children actively engaged in an activity. Your child's doctor needs to be contacted and likely will establish guidelines for you to follow.

1. What is the cause of this condition?
Causes include cardiac-related problems associated with the central (autonomic) nervous system, often brought on by various stimuli such as pain, fear, and other undesirable emotions. Rarer causes include cardiac arrhythmia (heart murmurs) and seizures.

2. Can this condition cause any long-term problems?
This depends on the diagnosis made.

3. What tests need to be performed to establish the cause?

Patient history and, at times, an electrocardiogram (EKG) or electroencephalogram (EEG) may be beneficial. If the problems persist and these tests are normal, then closed-circuit TV EEG monitoring of the patient in attempt to capture a fainting event would be recommended.

4. What safeguards do I need to employ to prevent it from happening again?

Your child should avoid the events that cause the fainting to occur, if those events are known. Often, however, this is not the case.

5. If fainting does occur, what steps do I take to ensure that my child will not be injured?

Avoid dangerous situations, plus educate your child in what to do if one of these episodes occurs.

6. Are there any medicines that we could use that would be of help?

This will depend on the diagnosis made.

7. Do we need to consult with a specialist, such as a cardiologist or neurologist?

If the symptoms cannot be easily explained, a cardiac and/or neurological workup is necessary.

8. What signs should I look for that would indicate I need to contact you?

If there is any prolonged episode of loss of consciousness, you should contact your doctor immediately.

9. When do you wish to see my child again regarding this condition?

Once a diagnosis is established and the patient placed on medication, we normally follow up with him or her in two to three months.

STEVEN L. LINDER, MD
Neurology

FIFTH DISEASE

Definition: An infectious skin disease characterized by reddened cheeks and lacy, flat, pink lesions on the surfaces of the body and extremities.

Author's Comment: The most important fact to know about this condition is that once the rash appears the child is no longer contagious. The contagious period takes place before the onset of the rash. The rash itself will usually disappear in two to three weeks, and the child may participate in normal activities during this period of time.

1. What causes this condition, and how did my child contract it?

Fifth disease is caused by a virus called parvovirus B19. It is a very common viral infection, contracted from another person with the infection. Many people with the infection have very mild symptoms and never see a physician for it. It can cause mild fever and headache and muscle aches for a few days. Several days later (often one to two weeks or more) the child may develop a rash that looks like a lace pattern on the body, and the cheeks may become red and look like they have been slapped. The child often does not feel ill by the time the rash comes on.

2. Is it contagious and, if so, for how long?

Fifth disease is contagious mainly before the rash comes out, so that by the time a person is recognized to have fifth disease, he or she is usually not contagious.

3. What complications can develop as a result of it?

Most persons have no complications from fifth disease. Adults may get arthritis (usually temporary), and immune-deficient persons may get other complications related to blood cell production. The most serious complication occurs if a pregnant woman gets fifth disease during pregnancy, especially in the first half of pregnancy. In this case, it can (in approximately 5 percent of cases) cause something called fetal hydrops that can result in death of the fetus.

4. How long will the rash last, and what other symptoms can occur?

The rash usually lasts for two to three weeks but may come and go for months. There are usually no other symptoms, but adults can have joint pain and swelling (arthritis) for prolonged periods of time.

5. What is the treatment, and what restrictions need to be imposed?

There is no treatment to get rid of the infection. It will go away on its own. No restrictions need to be imposed if the child feels well.

6. How long is the disorder contagious, and when can normal activities be resumed?

By the time the rash is recognized and the disease is diagnosed, the child is not contagious; the most contagious period is before the rash starts. Normal activities can be resumed as soon as the child feels up to them.

7. What dangers does this disease pose for people who have been exposed?

The main risk is to pregnant women and immune-deficient persons, as discussed in question #3.

8. What kind of follow-up will be needed?

None, unless your child seems to be developing a complication, such as arthritis.

GREGORY R. ISTRE, MD
Infectious Diseases

FLU
(Influenza)

Definition: An acute respiratory illness characterized
by congestion, sore throat, reddened eyes,
dry cough, fever, chills, and achiness.

Author's Comment: This condition causes doctors' offices to be
packed during the winter months and accounts for many school
absences. Fortunately, the flu vaccine offers good protection against
the common strains of flu each year and has little side effects. For
those who are unlucky enough to contract the flu, there are now new
medicines that can shorten the course of this illness, if started early.

1. What causes this condition, and how did my child contract it?
Flu (influenza) is caused by one of the influenza viruses. Influenza is
usually acquired from another person directly or indirectly.

2. What is its normal expected course?
The initial symptoms of influenza typically include fever, chills,
malaise, loss of appetite, headache, and, sometimes, muscle pain.

Later, sore throat, nasal congestion, and cough appear. Uncomplicated disease usually resolves without specific therapy within approximately seven days, but cough and malaise may linger.

3. Is it contagious, and how is it spread?

Influenza is highly contagious and is spread from person to person by droplets generated by coughing or sneezing or via direct contact with contaminated surfaces.

4. How long is the condition contagious, and when can my child resume activities?

The contagious period can vary significantly. In general, however, a child is considered contagious from twenty-four hours before the onset of symptoms until seven days after the symptoms begin. A child may resume activities as able.

5. What tests need to be done to more fully establish the diagnosis?

During seasonal epidemics, a diagnosis of influenza is often based on a child's symptoms and signs. Viral testing on secretions taken with a swab from the back of the nose can confirm the diagnosis.

6. Is there any treatment that can be done to shorten the course of the disease or make it less severe?

Several antiviral medications are available for the treatment of influenza. In general, treatment shortens the duration of illness to by one to two days, but only if started soon after symptoms begin.

7. Are there any potential side effects from the proposed treatment?

As with any medication, the drugs effective against influenza can have adverse effects. Depending on the particular agent, the most common side effects may include nausea and vomiting; nervousness, anxiety, or lightheadedness; and cough or breathing difficulties.

8. What symptoms or signs should I look for in my child that would necessitate my calling you back?

Reasons to call back include prolonged or recurrent fever, severe muscle pain, breathing difficulty, confusion or difficulty awakening your child, or any other symptoms of concern.

9. When do you wish to see my child again regarding this condition?

Typically, no specific follow-up is necessary.

STUART W. EHRETT, MD
Infectious Diseases

FOOD ALLERGY

Definition: An adverse reaction of the body to a food caused by an allergic mechanism.

Author's Comment: So many symptoms a child might be experiencing are attributed to food allergies—far more than actually exist. There is much myth and folklore associated with food allergy. It is important that you voice your concerns or suspicions in this area with your pediatrician.

1. What are the symptoms of food allergy?
Food allergy occurs when the body's system recognizes a food as a "foreign substance" and makes an allergic reaction to that food. The most common symptom of an allergic reaction to food is hives. Food allergy may also be a contributor to eczema. More serious food allergy reactions can cause sneezing, wheezing, cough, shortness of breath, swelling of the mouth, tongue or eyes, sudden quietness, vomiting, or diarrhea. Serious food allergy reactions can cause death. Most of the time, however, there is another cause for these symptoms.

It is important to distinguish food allergy from food intolerance. Food intolerance is a reaction to a food that is not caused by allergy. Examples of common food intolerances are insomnia caused by coffee; excessive gas caused by beans; or sneezing, runny nose, and watery eyes caused by hot peppers. In children, abdominal pain, diarrhea or vomiting, or rashes that are neither hives nor eczema may be caused by food intolerance.

2. How do I know if my child is allergic to a food?

Most of the time, a food allergy reaction will occur within one hour of eating the food or less. Food allergy does not come and go. If your child has an allergy to a food, the symptoms of the food allergy reaction will occur every time the food is eaten. Often, the same reaction will occur each time the food is eaten, but sometimes the reaction gets worse each time there is exposure to the food.

Food allergy seldom causes runny nose or stuffiness without some other reaction. Allergy symptoms (like runny nose or stuffiness) and asthma symptoms (like cough and wheeze) that do not get obviously worse right after eating are not caused by food allergy.

3. What is the value of food allergy testing?

Food allergy testing by skin test or blood test, like every other medical test, must be combined with a careful history to be useful. Because of the possibility of false-positive and false-negative tests, the results are only meaningful when interpreted together with the history of the reaction. Food allergy testing is best used to confirm the suspicion of food allergy based on reactions that have occurred. Knowing your child's history, the physician interpreting the test should be able to predict your child's risk of a severe food allergy reaction. Testing is often helpful in ruling out food allergy.

The most reliable food testing method is called a food challenge. In a food challenge, increasing amounts (beginning with a very small amount) of the suspect food are given every twenty to thirty minutes under careful medical supervision. The procedure is continued until the child has consumed the equivalent of a full portion of the food, such as 8 ounces of milk or 2 teaspoons of peanut butter. If there is no reaction during the challenge, the child is not allergic to that food. Food challenges are useful in the diagnosis of both food allergy and food intolerance.

4. What are elimination diets?

When there is suspicion that one or more foods are causing a problem, your doctor may recommend eliminating one or more foods from your child's diet. Elimination diets should last at least seven but not more than fourteen days. Because most children who are allergic to a food are allergic to only one or two foods, very limited diets are rarely needed. Because severely restricting a child's diet may lead to serious nutritional deficiencies, elimination diets should be short term and well planned to answer the question about a particular food.

If the symptoms disappear during the elimination diet, it *may* mean that the eliminated food caused the problem. The only way to confirm that the food is causing the problem is to reintroduce the food into the diet and reproduce the problems. This can only be done at home if the food is suspected to be a cause of minor problems such as diarrhea, hives, eczema, or runny nose and there has never been a serious reaction. If a food reaction has caused swelling of the mouth or eyes, sneezing, wheezing, coughing, or sudden quietness, the challenge should be done in a controlled medical setting where the doctor is prepared to take care of a life-threatening emergency.

5. What is the treatment for food allergy?

The only treatment for food allergy is to completely avoid the food that causes the problem.

6. What about rotation diets?

Rotation diets are based on the idea that eating a food for several days or more causes a reaction when eating the food once does not. There is no medical evidence that food allergy responds to rotation diets.

7. Can a food allergy be outgrown?

About 90 percent of children who are milk allergic at age one are no longer milk allergic at age three. There are no similar statistics for eggs, soy, or wheat but, in most children, these food allergies are often outgrown as well.

Allergies to peanuts, nuts that grow on trees (pecans, cashews, etc.), fish and shellfish are seldom outgrown. It is never safe to assume that a food allergy has been outgrown. If your child has had a serious reaction to a food, challenge testing as described in question #3 should be done before the food is reintroduced.

8. What should I do if my child has an allergic reaction to food?

If you think your child is having an allergic reaction to a food and the only symptom is a rash, you may give an antihistamine such as Benadryl and call your doctor.

If you think your child is having an allergic reaction to a food and the symptoms are sneezing, wheezing, coughing, and swelling of the eyes or mouth, or your child suddenly becomes very quiet, you must go to the nearest hospital emergency room. This may be a sign of anaphylaxis, a life-threatening allergic reaction.

9. If I have been told that my child is allergic to many foods, what can I feed him or her?

In a large study of children with proven food allergy, more than 90 percent of the children were allergic to only one or two foods. It is rare for a person to be allergic to many foods. A positive allergy blood test or skin test does not necessarily mean that your child is actually allergic to that food. False-positive reactions occur. These tests need to be interpreted with your child's history of food reactions. The only way to truly prove a food allergy is by doing a food challenge test.

If your child is allergic to many foods, you should work with your allergist, perhaps with the help of a nutritionist, to design an acceptable diet that is nutritionally adequate.

10. What are the resources to help maintain good nutrition and a normal life despite the food allergy?

The best place to start is with the Food Allergy and Anaphylaxis Network. This outstanding organization was started by the parent of a child with food allergy and has grown to be a major supporter of food allergy education and research. You can get help from their website, http://www.foodallergy.org/, phone (800) 929–4040, or you can write to them at 11781 Lee Jackson Hwy., Suite 160, Fairfax, VA 22033–3309.

11. My child is allergic to peanuts. Can I send him to school?

Dealing with food allergy in daycare or school requires close cooperation between the parents, teachers, and school officials. There should be a written policy on peanut products. Some schools have declared themselves "peanut free." What is appropriate for your child will depend on the child's age and ability to participate in avoiding peanuts. For example, most eight-year-olds can learn to ask about ingredients and refuse suspect foods; three-year-olds cannot.

RICHARD L. WASSERMAN, MD
Allergy and Immunology

FOREIGN BODY ASPIRATION

Definition: The breathing in of a foreign body into the respiratory tract.

Author's Comment: This is a frightening experience when it occurs to your child, and if the child does not cough up the foreign body on his or her own, it requires emergency action. One-year-olds should not be given popcorn, peanuts, unpeeled grapes, or unpeeled hot dogs, as these are common foods that infants can choke on and aspirate.

1. What are the problems created by this condition?

Foreign bodies in the airway may threaten life and produce severe lung damage. Aspiration can be accompanied by sudden violent coughing, gagging, wheezing, vomiting, cyanosis (turning blue), and apnea (not breathing). If the object is small and not obstructive, these reactions may be less dramatic. Patients can have an annoying cough and wheeze with respiratory distress. The object may obstruct only one part of the lung and cause overexpansion or underexpansion with atelectasis (partial collapse of the lung). Some foreign bodies such as seeds and nuts contain oils that can be very irritating to the airway, whereas small plastic parts (Legos, doll shoes) are much less irritating, and reactions may be subtler.

2. How dangerous is it?

Depending on the degree of the obstruction and the sharpness of object, there can be significant harm to the child. Respiratory distress can occur.

3. How do we plan to remove the foreign body, and is there any urgency to do it?

In general, it is best to remove the foreign body as soon as possible to reduce complications. Chest X rays or CT scans are often not helpful in making the diagnosis as they do not rule out a foreign body aspiration.

Foreign bodies in the airway of a child are best removed by bronchoscopy (usually done with a rigid bronchoscope) under general anesthesia. The modern bronchoscope comes in many sizes and allows for safe and efficient mechanical ventilation. It can provide a channel to insert special forceps to manipulate and retrieve the foreign body. If one is unsure if an airway foreign body is present, a flexible bronchoscopy may be done first.

4. Are there any dangers in attempting to get the foreign body out?

The usual reported complications are damage to lips, teeth, and gums; damage to the airway wall that may result in bleeding; infection; or pneumothorax (collapsed lung). Fortunately, in the hands of an experienced bronchoscopist (usually an otolaryngologist or pediatric surgeon) these complications are rare. There is also the danger that the object cannot be removed, despite several attempts, necessitating a thoracotomy (an open operation), but this is very rare. Following removal of a foreign body from the lower airway, there can be swelling of the vocal cord area due to manipulation or contact with chemicals in the foreign body. Steroids are often given postoperatively.

5. Should we consult a specialist and, if so, when?

A pediatric surgeon, otolaryngologist (ENT) or pediatric pulmonologist (lung specialist) should be contacted whenever an airway foreign body is suspected. If the aspiration was witnessed and the child is showing symptoms, you should immediately contact your pediatrician and proceed to the nearest emergency room.

6. Has any permanent damage occurred as a result of the foreign body?

Generally speaking, when the object has not been in the airway for long or has not moved, there is essentially no permanent damage to the lungs. The longer a foreign body is down the airway or the more irritating it is, the more likely there can be some sort of scarring of the airway wall. Chronic aspiration occurs when an irritating object, such as a nut, is lodged in the airway for weeks to months, possibly producing scarring and permanent damage.

7. How can we prevent this from happening again?

The best prevention in young children is to avoid foods that can easily be choked on. These include seeds, nuts, popcorn, unpeeled hot dogs, and other large pieces of meats. Vigilance in feeding young kids and preventing older kids from choking (chewing and choking on pen caps is common) is key. Early medical help prevents most long-term complications.

PETER N. SCHOCHET, MD
Pulmonary

GANGLION

Definition: A cyst on the outside lining of the joint
or the outside lining of the tendon.

Author's Comment: These lumps that children develop over bony
structures are totally safe but at times can be painful. When one
appears, the hope is that it will disappear on its own, but if it does not,
the child may need to see a skilled orthopedist (bone doctor).

1. What causes this condition to occur?
A ganglion is a cyst or fluid collection on the outside lining of the
joint or the outside lining of the tendon. Most of the time there is no
good reason why this condition occurs. This condition can occur after
injuries or infections. Sometimes it can occur along with the development of childhood rheumatism or arthritis.

2. Is it dangerous, and can it develop into something else?
It is not dangerous, and it cannot develop into something else. A
ganglion cyst is truly benign, and unless there are symptoms of pain,
no intervention is necessary.

3. Do any tests need to be performed to further aid in the diagnosis or treatment?

Yes. A physical examination often reveals a typical feel or appearance to a cyst. To confirm a ganglion cyst, there are three options: (1) ultrasound can confirm the fluid-filled cyst, and, if so, this requires no intervention; (2) an MRI can also show if the bump is fluid filled or cystic in nature, but this is a more expensive test compared to the ultrasound. (In very young children, an MRI requires the child to be completely still and sedation is used, whereas with an ultrasound these are not needed.); and (3) a needle aspiration can be done for fluid drainage. The fluid may reveal the certain appearance of a ganglion cyst.

4. What are the options for treatment of this condition, and do we need to see an orthopedist (bone doctor)?

Once the diagnosis of a ganglion cyst is confirmed, no intervention is necessary if there are no symptoms. This is a benign condition that will never become cancerous. If there are symptoms, the cyst can be drained with a needle. Removing the fluid and flattening the sac may help. If the cyst returns, it can be aspirated again. After a few aspirations, another option would be to aspirate the cyst and then inject steroid material into the area to try to flatten the cyst.

The cyst can also be surgically removed. There is no absolute guarantee that surgical removal will keep it from returning. In fact, there is 20 percent to 50 percent chance that a ganglion cyst can recur following surgical removal. For a noncancerous, benign cyst, really no treatment is needed, and surgical excision typically is the last measure that should be offered. You are basically trading a bump for a scar, and there is a high chance of recurrence.

5. What limitations does this condition impose upon my child's activities?

None. Your child can be as active as the comfort allows. Typically a ganglion cyst causes no discomfort, and again, if there is discomfort associated with the cyst, further investigation of the area near the joint would be recommended.

6. What kind of follow-up is needed at your office concerning this condition?

If there is no change in the appearance of the cyst and, more importantly, if there are no symptoms, such as pain, discomfort, or inability to do things, then no further follow-up is needed for this benign condition. The natural history of a ganglion cyst is that it is intermittent. Some activities may increase the size of the cyst, and later it decreases with rest. If your child has no symptoms, there is no need for further follow-up.

W. BARRY HUMENIUK, MD
Orthopedics

HAIR LOSS (Alopecia)

Author's Comment: It is important that your child sees the doctor to establish the cause for the hair loss. Most of the time the hair loss is temporary or correctable, but at times, it is progressive, leading to much alarm and anxiety on the part of parent and child.

1. What causes this condition?

There are many types of hair loss, and they occur for a variety of reasons. Some types are congenital (present since birth). In these children, the cause of hair loss is usually a genetic (inherited) condition or a structural abnormality of the hair. It is how the child's hair is made—he or she is born that way.

Other types of hair loss are acquired later in life. There are many types of acquired hair loss, and the cause varies with each type. Some hair loss follows scalp infections, such as tinea capitis (ringworm). Other types of hair loss are the result of skin conditions (such as lupus) that cause inflammation of the scalp, or other medical conditions, like thyroid disease or poor nutrition. One of the most common types of hair loss in children is alopecia areata. This is an autoimmune condition of unknown cause in which inflammation develops around the hairs causing them to fall out. Also common is telogen effluvium in which the hair is shed after a stressful event, such as a prolonged high fever or surgery. This is the same type of hair loss that women often experience after having a baby.

Hair loss can also be due to certain medications, the most common being chemotherapy drugs. Some people incorrectly believe that cancer makes people's hair fall out—the truth is that hair loss in cancer patients is due to the treatment, not the disease.

Hair loss can be due to trauma to the scalp. This can occur due to prolonged pressure on the scalp (for example, if the head is in the same position during a very long surgery or hospitalization) or if the hair is styled too tightly in braids or ponytails for a long period of time. Chemical treatments such as harsh perms can damage the hair and make it fall out. Lastly, some hair loss is self-inflicted by hair pulling. Hair pulling can be a simple habit in some children, but in others it may be a sign of deeper psychological issues.

2. What tests should be done to establish the cause?

Many types of hair loss can be diagnosed with a few well-directed questions and a good physical examination alone. If a child has little to no hair from birth or if his or her hair does not grow (such that he or she never needs a haircut) then he or she likely has a congenital, inherited, or structural defect of the hair. The type of structural defects can be determined by having your doctor, usually a dermatologist, examine your child's hair under the microscope.

Children who have completely normal hair growth for the first few years of life then lose hair suddenly or in patches usually have one of the acquired types of hair loss. If a child shows signs of thyroid disease or has a family history of this, then thyroid levels should be checked. If a nutritional problem, like severe anemia due to low iron, is suspected, then checking a blood count can be helpful. Children who have evidence of a bacterial or fungal infection of the scalp may need cultures performed.

Occasionally a skin biopsy may be needed to confirm the cause of hair loss. In general, there are no specific tests that need to be done in every child with hair loss, and many children will require no tests at all. When tests are needed to make or confirm a diagnosis, they should be tailored to the individual child's history and exam findings.

3. Is the condition contagious?

Most forms of hair loss are not contagious. The exception would be hair loss due to fungal (ringworm) or bacterial scalp infections.

4. Will it get worse?

The congenital or inherited forms of hair loss tend to stay the same, but some forms may show improvement with age. Hair loss due to an underlying medical or skin disorder, medications, hair pulling, infection, or continued trauma to the hair or scalp will continue to worsen until the underlying cause is identified and remedied. Alopecia areata can worsen progressively, and some children may permanently lose all of their hair, but more often the areas of hair loss will come and go over time. Alopecia areata is unique in that the hair may grow back spontaneously in some children, even without treatment.

5. Could there be a psychological cause for this disorder?

Although people commonly believe that hair loss is due to "stress," this is not usually the case. Nevertheless, self-inflicted hair loss in children who pull their own hair out can be a sign of underlying psychological problems, such as depression. It may be a subconscious cry for help. Nevertheless, children who pull their hair out will often deny doing it and may hide the evidence. Some children even eat the hair that they have pulled out.

If your child has experienced a traumatic event, such as the loss of a parent, or if he or she shows signs of psychological problems or depression, then he or she may benefit from consultation with a child psychiatrist. Signs of depression include inability to sleep, loss of appetite, lack of interest in friends or activities, or poor school performance.

6. Will the hair grow back, and, if so, over what period of time?

For most acquired types of hair loss, once the underlying cause of the hair loss is treated then the hair usually grows back. The hair grows approximately 1 centimeter a month, so noticeable hair regrowth typically takes 2 to 3 months. In children with telogen effluvium, the hair usually returns slowly over a period of four to six months.

For hair loss due to infections, inflammatory skin conditions or trauma to the scalp, the scalp may need some time to recover, so improvement is slower and may not be noted for six to twelve months. During this time it is important to treat the hair as gently as possible and avoid damaging hair treatments such as perms, chemical straighteners, or styling using high-heat styling devices. If the scalp inflammation was severe or prolonged, then scarring may occur; the hair loss may be permanent in these areas.

7. Assuming the hair grows back, will it be of the same thickness, color, and consistency as before?

Sometimes the new hair growth is more fine or coarse than the old hair. It can also be a little lighter or darker in color. In alopecia areata, the initial hair regrowth may be white. In cases of telogen effluvium or if there was trauma or prolonged inflammation of the scalp skin, the hair that grows back may not be as thick as before. Over time, the color and texture of the hair usually returns to normal, but not always.

8. Are there any medicines to be used and, if so, for how long? What are the potential side effects from these medications?

The treatment depends on the cause of the hair loss. For most congenital, inherited, or structural hair disorders, no treatment is available. If there is a bacterial or fungal infection, then oral antibiotics (for two weeks, sometimes longer) or antifungal medications (for two to four months) are used. These medications are usually well tolerated, but stomach upset or allergic reactions can occur. Oral antifungals can affect the liver (the newer antifungals moreso than the old ones), and they may interact with other oral medications.

Inflammatory scalp conditions usually respond well to topical steroid treatment; this therapy may need to be ongoing. Topical steroids when used as directed are generally quite safe, but since more potent topical steroids are usually required for scalp conditions, thinning of the skin over time is possible. As a result, periodic follow-up with your doctor is recommended so that he or she can monitor for any side effects. Topical minoxidil liquid is helpful for some types of hair loss but should only be used with a doctor's supervision in children. Side effects include blood pressure changes, skin irritation, and increased hair growth on the forehead (if the medication is accidentally applied there).

For hair pulling due to psychological issues, psychiatric counseling and/or medications may be needed. For alopecia areata, steroids (topical, oral, or injected) are usually the first line of treatment, but anthralin cream, contact sensitization therapy, or minoxidil can be used if your child does not respond to steroids. These treatments may need to be continued for months, since new areas of hair loss often continue to appear off and on. Steroids injected into the scalp lesions can cause skin thinning. Oral steroids can cause weight gain, moodiness, increased blood pressure, bone thinning, growth delay, and acne. Giving the steroids at once-monthly intervals rather than daily or taking scheduled breaks from the medication can help to limit these side effects. Anthralin and contact sensitization both cause skin irritation and redness.

9. Do we need to see a specialist for this condition?

Some forms of hair loss look very similar and can be difficult to distinguish. If the diagnosis is not certain, then your child may require the help of a dermatologist. Also, if your child is not responding to therapy as expected or if he or she has significant inflammation and is at risk for scarring or permanent hair loss, your child may benefit from a visit to a specialist. A specialist can also be helpful in diagnosing more rare types of hair loss, such as structural or congenital hair abnormalities, and may feel more comfortable using oral medications or more aggressive treatments than a nonspecialist.

10. When do you wish to see my child again regarding this disorder?

This depends on the type of hair loss. For congenital types of hair loss, no follow-up may be needed since we do not have a good way to treat most of these conditions. For alopecia areata, your child should be seen again in three months, since new hair growth can usually be seen in this amount of time, but more frequent visits may be needed if your child is receiving oral steroid or contact sensitization therapy. For scalp infections, follow-up in two to four weeks is recommended to be sure that the infection is clearing with treatment.

K. ROBIN CARDER, MD
Dermatology

HAND, FOOT, AND MOUTH SYNDROME

Definition: A condition characterized by reddened blister-like eruptions of the hands, feet, and mouth.

Author's Comment: This viral syndrome gets better on its own but sometimes causes considerable discomfort, especially if there are mouth lesions present. However, not all children with this disease develop lesions in the mouth.

1. What causes this condition, and how did my child contract it?

One of the most common causes of mouth ulcers in children under three years of age is hand, foot, and mouth disease, which is usually caused by infection with coxsackie virus. Painful blister-like elevations (vesicles) and ulcers can develop on the tongue and back of the mouth. A tender skin rash may also occur characteristically on the hands, feet, buttock, and groin. Sore throat and low-grade fever may sometimes occur. The infection is spread by contact with an infected person's secretions, such as saliva and stool.

2. Is it contagious and, if so, for how long?

The virus is most contagious during the first week of disease, but it can continue to spread for several weeks after symptoms of the illness have resolved. Handwashing is essential to prevent spread to others in the household, particularly with diaper changes.

3. What is the natural course for this condition, and what complications can occur?

The condition typically resolves by itself. The most common complication is dehydration caused by mouth pain and decreased oral intake.

4. Is there any treatment that needs to be employed?

There is no antiviral therapy recommended for this disease.

5. What type of restrictions need to be imposed on my child's activities?

Your child should be kept out of child care or school until the fever is gone and mouth sores have healed.

6. How long does this illness last?

The illness usually lasts for about a week.

7. What can I do to make my child feel better?

Supportive care with over-the-counter pain relievers may help with pain control. Encourage your child to drink plenty of fluids and eat popsicles.

8. When do you wish to see my child again for this condition?

Unless there are complications, your child usually does not need to be seen again for this illness. You should contact your doctor if your child is not drinking enough. Occasionally children may need to be admitted to the hospital for rehydration with intravenous fluids.

WENDY CHUNG, MD
Infectious Diseases

HAY FEVER
(Allergic Rhinitis)

Definition: An allergic condition characterized by runny nose and watery eyes that is frequently chronic or seasonal.

Author's Comment: This condition seems to be occurring with greater frequency among children, possibly due to the increasing pollution in our environment. Fortunately, in recent years, scientists have found many good medicines that can control the symptoms and cause few side effects.

1. What causes this condition, and how did my child develop it?

Allergic rhinitis (commonly referred to as "allergies" or "hay fever") is a very common condition, occurring in approximately 20 percent of the general population. The well-known symptoms of runny nose, sneezing, and itchy, watery eyes occur immediately upon exposure to any number of airborne allergens that we are all exposed to, including dust mites, animal danders, molds, and pollen. There is nothing intrinsically harmful about these substances, except to those individuals who are genetically "wired" to make allergic antibodies to them.

Many of the symptoms of allergic rhinitis make this condition difficult to differentiate from viral upper respiratory infections (URIs), which are also very common in young children during the fall, winter, and spring months. Hayfever symptoms can be distinguished from URI symptoms if they occur with exposure to a known allergen (such as grandmother's cat); with the presence of itching and absence of fever; and if other allergic conditions in the child or in immediate family members exist. Because the development of an allergic sensitivity requires repeated exposure to an allergen, seasonal allergic rhinitis is very uncommon in children less than three years of age. However, year-round (or perennial) nasal allergy symptoms caused by airborne, indoor allergens may start during infancy.

2. What medicines should my child use to treat it?

There are several classes of medications used to prevent and treat the symptoms of allergic rhinitis. The most commonly prescribed medications are the antihistamines, which include well-known brands such as Benadryl, Claritin, Zyrtec, Xyzal, and Allegra. These medications work by blocking the histamine receptors found in the lining of the respiratory passages, thereby blunting the immediate symptoms of itching, sneezing, and runny nose. Antihistamines are often given as needed for relief of allergic symptoms. Antihistamines given as a preventative, prior to an anticipated allergen exposure may help prevent allergic symptoms. Note that antihistamines are not very effective for relief of nasal congestion associated with allergic rhinitis.

Oral decongestant medications, such as pseudoephedrine, are found both alone (e.g., Sudafed) and in combination with antihistamines in many over-the-counter and prescription allergy medications.

Additional medications that are used to prevent or control chronic nasal allergy symptoms include medicated nasal sprays and leukotriene-modifying agents. The medicated nasal sprays include Nasalcrom, Astelin, and topical corticosteroids (many brands, including Flonase, Nasonex, Nasacort, Nasarel, and Rhinocort).

3. What are the side effects of these medicines?

Older antihistamines such as Benadryl and medications containing chlorpheniramine and brompheniramine cause some degree of sedation at usual doses. This side effect may help an uncomfortable child get a good night's sleep but is clearly undesirable in terms of daytime cognitive functioning. These antihistamines can occasionally cause irritability or wild behavior in young children. Such side effects usually resolve four to six hours after taking the dose. Newer antihistamines (e.g., Claritin, Zyrtec, Xyzal, and Allegra) carry a much lower potential for sedation and thus rarely cause unwanted antihistamine side effects.

Oral decongestant medications such as pseudoephedrine may cause short-term side effects of irritability or insomnia. Medicated nasal sprays may cause irritation of the nasal membranes and, less commonly, nosebleeds. The risk of nosebleeds can be reduced somewhat by directing the tip of the nasal spray away from the nasal septum. Corticosteroid nasal sprays are not known to cause growth retardation or other systemic steroid effects.

4. Is there anything we can do in our home environment to make this condition better?

While identification and avoidance of the offending allergen(s) is considered the first step in treating an allergic condition, this is not always possible or practical. For children who are found to be allergic to dust mites, special encasements for the mattress and pillows can be very effective for reducing chronic nasal allergy symptoms. Because dust mites thrive in relative humidity above 50 percent, using a humidifier may actually cause more harm than good.

Children who are allergic to animal danders will benefit from removing the offending animal(s) from the home. However, one should understand that without thorough cleaning of the household fabrics, the dander can linger and cause ongoing symptoms for up to six months after the pet departs. Note that air duct cleaning has not been shown to help people with allergies; instead, attention should be paid to the routine care of the air conditioning system, including regular changing of the filters.

Finally, tobacco smoke, which is known to irritate respiratory passages (and lingers long after the cigarette is extinguished), should be excluded from the home and car at all times.

5. How long will this condition last?

Unfortunately, many children who are genetically predisposed to develop allergies will continue to acquire more allergic sensitivities through their first decade of life. Nasal allergy symptoms can be bothersome through all decades of life. While the course and severity of the allergic condition is unpredictable, a pattern of severe allergy symptoms usually indicates similar problems down the line.

6. What complications can my child develop from this condition?

The spectrum of complications resulting from untreated nasal allergies is broad, including recurrent ear and sinus infections, bronchial asthma, dental misalignment necessitating braces, and sleep disturbance leading to learning and/or behavioral problems.

7. Is this an allergic condition, and, if so, how long should we wait to see an allergist?

The symptoms of allergic rhinitis may be difficult to distinguish from those of viral URIs in very young children. If your child has other allergic features (such as infantile eczema) or a strong family history of allergies, chances are better than not that the chronic nasal symptoms are allergic. Regardless of the child's age, if the rhinitis symptoms do not respond satisfactorily to a trial of allergy medications or are complicated by recurrent infections or asthma, referral to an allergist is recommended for additional evaluation and management.

8. When do I call you back regarding my child's progress?

You should call if the allergy symptoms are not clearly improving within one week after starting medications, sooner if your child's condition is worsening or you observe medication side effects.

9. Will you need to see my child again regarding this condition?

If the allergy symptoms are manageable with medications, the problem and its treatment will be reviewed at your child's annual wellness visit. If the allergies are complicated by recurrent infections or asthma, follow-up visits should be scheduled twice a year to review the child's progress and consider additional interventions.

ROBERT W. SUGERMAN, MD
Allergy and Immunology

HEADACHES

Author's Comment: This is a very common complaint among children. It is important that you consult your child's doctor to rule out any serious underlying condition if the headaches persist or occur with significant frequency.

1. What is the cause of my child's headaches?

There are multiple causes of headaches—most are benign. A thorough history, physical examination, neurological examination, and headache examination is necessary to make sure the headaches are not serious. The most common recurrent headache is migraine. Sinus headaches are usually at the nasal bridge and not associated with classic symptoms of migraine, which are light and noise sensitivity and abdominal discomfort.

2. Are we sure that they are not a symptom of something more serious going on in the head?

We become concerned if the patient has early morning vomiting with headaches. There is no classical history that definitely identifies a brain tumor or other space-occupying lesions, but early morning headaches with vomiting are often suspicious. Keep records of headaches and avoid excessive intake of caffeine, establish good sleeping habits (eight to nine hours per night), and ensure that your child is eating appropriately without skipping meals, as well as drinking lots of fluids, especially when it is excessively hot. These simple procedures can often prevent routine headaches.

3. Are there more tests that need to be performed to better define the cause of this disorder?

If the patient does not respond to treatment or has abnormalities on neurological examination, your doctor may want to obtain an MRI scan of the brain.

4. What medicine(s) should we use to treat the headaches?

Over-the-counter medications, such as ibuprofen and acetaminophen, can be helpful. If there is no clinical improvement then, your doctor might consider the "triptan" drugs such as Imitrex, Maxalt, Zomig, Relpax, and Axert. None of these drugs have been formally approved by the Food and Drug Administration (FDA) for the use in children and adolescents seventeen years of age or younger, but they are frequently used by pediatric neurologists and are effective.

5. What are the potential side effects of these medicines?

Over-the-counter medications for standard use have no acute complications. Long-term use of acetaminophen can cause injury to the liver. Long-term use of ibuprofen can cause gastrointestinal difficulties as well as kidney disease. Triptans may have "triptan" side effects, which include tingling sensations in the throat, neck, shoulders, but in general more serious cardiac problems are extremely rare.

6. Is it important to have my child's eyes checked?

Normally, the eyes should be checked only if the patient complains of a specific, reproducible visual problem or if the headache is exacerbated with reading. If the patient has similar complaints and has recurrent, uncontrolled headaches and the physician cannot see the optic discs (where the optic nerve enters the retina) adequately, then further examination may be necessary.

7. What symptoms do I look for to make sure the condition is not evolving into something more serious?

Signs to look for would be a change in the headache patterns and severity as well as early morning vomiting, abnormal walking, unusual visual complaints, and altered mental status.

8. How long do I wait to call you back if the symptoms persist?

Generally, if the headache lasts greater than three days, a physician should be contacted, especially with a new, uncontrolled, and unprovoked headache. If the patient has recurrent headaches and a normal neurological examination, he or she should be seen for follow-up in two to three months. The family should keep detailed records regarding the headaches and the amount of medication used.

9. When would we need to see a neurologist?

A consultation should be sought with a neurologist for specific diagnosis and a treatment plan, especially if the headaches are not controlled with standard medications. Most pediatricians still feel uncomfortable with using the triptan drugs for acute management and often do not like to start daily preventative medications, with the exception of Periactin. If the patient is having one headache per week or one to two severe headaches per month and missing an excessive amount of school, then consultation should be considered.

10. When do you wish to see my child again regarding this condition?

Normally we see the patient back in three months for repeat examination and for answering the family's as well as the child's questions and to make sure no further evaluation is necessary. A diary is extremely important for looking for specific patterns as well as for documenting clinical response to medicines used.

STEVEN L. LINDER, MD
Neurology

HEAD ASYMMETRY

Definition: **Irregularly shaped skull.**

Author's Comment: Some of these conditions are mild and may be more noticeable to the parents than they are to the casual observer. Nevertheless, the condition should be followed by your child's doctor and, if severe, may warrant further evaluation and treatment.

1. What causes this condition to occur?

The skull is very soft in infants. When they stay in one position over long periods of time and repetitively, the brain grows in the direction of least resistance. The skull shape follows the growth of the brain. This leads to the common abnormal head shape with a protrusion on one side of the forehead, a flattening on the back of the head, and abnormal alignment of the ears. This change occurs over time and is very rarely present at birth. This particular head shape deformity is acquired and not related to genetic predisposition or maternal prenatal care.

Head shape deformities and asymmetries are very common. Most are not even noticeable by the everyday public. Some asymmetries run in families and are not considered to be an issue. However, in recent years, since the American Association of Pediatrics recommended that all children should sleep on their backs to reduce the incidence of sudden infant death, there has been a significant increase in the incidence of head shape deformities, most notably positional plagiocephaly. This is not a surgical disease in the vast majority of cases. The head shape change occurs because the child spends a significant time on his or her back, or with the head turned to one side, with a decrease in movement or position change. This does not just occur during sleep but also when children are placed in automatic swings, car seat carriers, or strollers for extended periods of time without changing their position.

2. Is there any brain damage associated with this condition?

No. There is no brain damage associated with positional or deformational head shape changes. That being said, children with neurological disorders, including brain damage, may have deformational head shape changes, but they are the result of the brain injury not the cause of it.

3. Are any diagnostic tests needed to be done to further define the problem?

The diagnosis of positional plagiocephaly is largely a clinical diagnosis. Sometimes, when the clinical exam is difficult, plain X rays of the skull can be taken to evaluate the presence or absence of open skull sutures, similar to looking at the growth plates of the joints in long bones. When the X rays are taken, you can see whether or not the sutures are open or closed. If one or more of the sutures is closed, the you are dealing with a different problem: craniosynostosis.

Some insurance companies may require that X rays be taken prior to a doctor's visit so that a definitive diagnosis can be made. A CAT scan is largely unnecessary except for severe cases where the plain X rays are not helpful. These should be ordered by the craniofacial specialist or neurosurgeon, due to the expense and the sedation risks required to perform the scan on infants.

4. What can be done to correct the deformity?

The key to successful treatment of the child is early diagnosis. If treatment begins before the age of four months, excellent results usually follow with the return of a normal head shape. Early treatment is defined as frequent position changes, such as not leaving the child in a swing or a car seat (except when driving) for more than thirty minutes at a time. If it is necessary to keep the child in one of these devices, his or her position should be changed frequently. Also, tummy time is recommended when the child is not being held, fed, or sleeping. All this entails is putting a blanket of the floor and the child on the blanket on his or her stomach. This stimulates improvements in neck strength and mobility as well as upper body strength and development. When the neck muscles are tight, physical therapy for neck range of motion is recommended. This can be done at the physical therapist's office at first and then continued on a regular basis at home by the parents. The vast majority of children can be treated this way.

Additional treatment can be obtained by the use of a headband or helmet. This is somewhat controversial as research on treatment outcomes and reliability of therapy are not well established. Evidence-based evaluations, or just looking at the results of hundreds of children treated with helmets and headbands, demonstrate significant improvement in head shape, if the treatment is begun before twelve months of age, especially if begun before six months. Many physicians reserve this therapy for the most severe cases or those that do not respond to the conservative treatment of position change, tummy time, and physical therapy.

5. What would happen if we just sit back and do nothing but observe the head as it grows?

The likelihood of the head returning to a more normal shape by two to three years of age is pretty high, but there is very little data to support this. However, if you look at the number of children who have head asymmetry as infants, and then the ones who have it at two to three years of age, the difference is astounding. I do not believe that all of the children with this deformity go to the doctor for treatment. If it did not correct on its own, we should be seeing a large volume of older children with asymmetric heads and faces. The fact is we see very few. In most cases, the asymmetry corrects itself without intervention. From experience, the cases that are unlikely to correct without therapy are the children with torticollis (neck muscle contraction), neurological problems, and severe asymmetries. These patients may require additional therapy with headbands or helmets.

6. Should we consider a physical therapist or a craniofacial surgeon to evaluate the condition and to determine if a corrective helmet is needed?

The pediatrician should make the diagnosis or refer you to a craniofacial or pediatric neurosurgeon for evaluation, diagnosis, and treatment. Some helmet companies advertise their own physical therapist who would recommend a helmet or banding therapy, but there is a conflict of interest here as well as a duplication of efforts. Instead, if the child visits the specialist physician first, time is saved, charges are reduced, and an evaluation and treatment plan is developed in one sitting.

Referrals should be made when the asymmetry is severe (i.e., affecting the face in addition to the head), if the child has torticollis (neck muscle contraction), or if there is something that is so concerning to the pediatrician that they want help. Once the diagnosis is made, the physician can decide what level of therapy is necessary. Most of the time, the treatment will include physical therapy, position changes, and tummy time.

7. When do you wish to see my child again for this condition?

The pediatrician follows this condition during routine checkups. If a craniofacial surgeon is consulted, the follow-up depends on what is decided at the initial evaluation. Often, if the child is placed on conservative therapy, he or she can be followed up in three months. If helmet therapy is started, the follow-up is performed after the therapy is completed or if another band or helmet is requested.

DAVID GENECOV, MD
Craniofacial Surgery

HEAD LICE

Definition: **Parasitic insects that infect the hair and scalp, causing reddened areas and itching.**

Author's Comment: This condition is repugnant to most parents. It exists at times in epidemic proportions, especially in schools and daycare centers. In some children, the condition is resistant to some of the conventional therapies, but your doctor will find a treatment that will kill even the most resistant of bugs.

1. What causes this condition, and how did my child contract it?

Head lice are very small insects that feed on small amounts of blood. They commonly cause an itchy infestation of the scalp, with small red bumps on the scalp, neck, and shoulders. Small tan eggs (nits) attach to hair shafts and hatch in about one to two weeks. Nits can look like dandruff but cannot be removed by shaking them off. Lice are spread by direct contact with an infected person, or with infected clothing or bedding.

2. What is the treatment, and how effective is it?

For children over two years of age, head lice can usually be effectively treated by using over-the-counter, medicated shampoo that is specifically formulated to kill lice. The treatment may need to be repeated in seven days. If the product still does not kill the lice, however, your doctor can prescribe a prescription drug for treating head lice. For two weeks, a fine-toothed comb can be used on wet hair, every few days, to physically remove the nits. Cutting the hair very short may also be helpful.

3. Are there any potential side effects of the treatment?

When used as directed, the topical treatments are generally well tolerated, with skin irritation and hypersensitivity being the most common side effects. The prescription medication malathion is highly flammable, and therefore should be used away from all heat sources, such as cigarettes and hair dryers.

4. How will I know if all the lice have been killed following treatment?

Medicated treatments are usually effective at killing the lice, but the itching may continue for a few days. Nits may still be seen in your child's hair after treatment, but the eggs may be empty. If nits are still found in the hair within a quarter inch of the scalp, however, they should be treated. A second shampoo treatment in seven to ten days is often recommended to make sure all nits have been killed.

5. What advice should be given to people who have been recently exposed to my child?

Watch for complaints of itching and scratching of the scalp. Examine those who have had close contact with infected persons every three to four days, checking for nits and lice on the scalp, behind the ears, and on the nape of the neck.

6. How contagious is this condition, and when is my child no longer contagious?

Head lice are very contagious, and not a sign of poor hygiene. Lice can survive up to thirty days on a person, and up to three days off the scalp. They are easily passed by close contact with an infected person, particularly within the same household. Teach your child not to share hats, scarves, combs, or brushes at school. All possibly contaminated items should be washed in hot water and soap, including clothing, bedding, hats, combs, brushes, and stuffed animals. Any unwashable items can be placed in a sealed bag for two weeks. Floors should be vacuumed, and furniture can be covered with plastic drop cloth for two weeks.

7. How much school should my child miss as a result of this condition?

Although children should not be sent home early from school because of discovery of head lice, the child should be treated before returning to school on the day following treatment. It is not necessary to require that a treated child be completely free of nits before returning to school or child care.

8. When do you wish to see my child again regarding this disorder?

You should contact your physician if there is still difficulty eradicating the lice after a treatment. Head lice can cause extreme itching but does not lead to serious medical problems. Scratching can cause secondary bacterial skin infections, which should be brought to the attention of your child's physician.

WENDY CHUNG, MD
Infectious Diseases

HEARING DEFICIT

Definition: **Diminished hearing.**

Author's Comment: This condition needs to be detected early and, if it persists, needs to be fully checked out and, if possible, corrected. It is thought by many that hearing problems in young infants left untreated can lead to learning differences later on. Fortunately, most hospital nurseries now screen their newborns to rule out hearing loss.

1. What causes this condition?

Hearing loss in children is due to many causes. The most common causes of hearing loss in children are conductive (CHL), while nerve deafness or sensorineural hearing loss (SNHL) is less common. Conductive hearing loss is typically due to ear infections or persistent fluid in the ear. Sensorineural hearing loss is typically due to an abnormality of the inner ear that affects the conversion of sound waves into nerve impulses.

304 1001 Healthy Baby Answers

2. Was my child born with this condition, or was it acquired?

As mentioned previously, conductive causes of hearing loss are most commonly due to ear infections. Less common causes may be damage to the eardrum or ear bones due to chronic ear infections. Birth defects affecting the ear bones or ear canal can cause CHL. Sensorineural hearing loss is usually present from birth and most often due to inherited causes. Exposure to loud noises, such as music played at high volumes, can result in SNHL. Other acquired causes of SNHL are exposure to certain intravenous antibiotics, trauma, and autoimmune disorders.

3. What tests need to be performed to further define the cause and severity?

In many states in the U.S., universal screening of newborns is done to detect congenital hearing loss. Typically children who fail screening are referred for either auditory brainstem response (ABR) or otoacoustic emission (OAE) testing. Both of these tests are electrophysiologic measures of hearing. While not as accurate as behavioral (sound booth) testing, ABR and OAE allow for testing of infants, toddlers, and other children with developmental delays who cannot respond to sound booth testing. If your child fails a screening test, he or she will be referred for more extensive testing. Infants and younger children may be tested with ABR or OAE; for older children, sound booth testing is done.

4. Is there any treatment for this disorder?

In general, conductive hearing loss is reversible, while sensorineural hearing loss is not. CHL due to ear infections may be treated medically (with antibiotics or allergy medications) or with surgery (placement of ear tubes into the eardrums). For chronic ear disorders affecting the ear bones or the eardrum, reconstructive surgery may be required. While no cures are available for SNHL, rehabilitative treatment is available. For profound hearing loss (complete nerve deafness), cochlear implantation is available. A cochlear implant converts sound waves to electrical impulses, which stimulate nerve endings of the cochlear (hearing) nerve. All hearing loss, whether CHL or SNHL, is treatable with hearing aids.

5. Is the condition correctable?

In general, conductive causes of hearing loss, such as middle ear fluid (otitis media), impacted earwax, and chronic conditions of the middle ear (such as cholesteatoma), can be treated surgically, and hearing can be restored. Nerve deafness is not correctable except by rehabilitation with either hearing aides or cochlear implantation if the hearing loss is profound.

6. Has my child's learning process been affected?

Hearing loss, whether conductive or sensorineural, may lead to learning or developmental delays. In younger children, speech delays may result. Hearing loss may also exacerbate delays in children who are already developmentally delayed. In school-age children, hearing loss can interfere with reading or spelling. Hearing loss at a young age, such as conductive hearing loss due to middle ear fluid, may contribute to problems with auditory processing in school-age children. Auditory processing disorders affect how a child hears and understands what is being said. This may lead to listening problems at school or in the home.

7. Does my child need to see an ear, nose, and throat (ENT) physician or an audiologist (hearing specialist)?

Your pediatrician will determine if a referral to an ENT physician is necessary. The ENT specialist along with an audiologist should examine children identified with a hearing loss to determine the exact nature and causes of a conductive hearing loss. Once the type and cause of hearing loss has been identified, treatment can be initiated.

8. When do you wish to see my child again for this condition?

Follow-up for hearing loss depends on the nature of the loss. For children with conductive hearing loss due to middle ear fluid, follow-up every four to six weeks is recommended until the condition has resolved, either with medical (antibiotics) or surgical treatment (placement of ear tubes). With sensorineural hearing loss, follow-up either annually or biannually is recommended once it has been determined the hearing loss has stabilized.

MICHAEL BIAVATI, MD
Otolaryngology

HEART MURMUR

Definition: **An abnormal heart sound.**

Author's Comment: Heart murmurs are very common in childhood. If they are of the "innocent" type, which means there is no structural abnormality, there is nothing to worry about. The organic type of murmur signifies some structural abnormality, which may be problematic for the child. Sometimes it is difficult for even the most skilled physician to be able to distinguish between the two with stethoscope alone. These children often need further investigation, sometimes from a pediatric cardiologist (heart specialist).

1. What causes this condition?

Heart murmurs occur in many children. The majority of heart murmurs are termed "innocent" heart murmurs. This simply means that the murmur is not caused by any kind of defect or abnormality with the heart. An innocent murmur simply means the normal flow of blood through the heart is being heard. Less commonly, a heart murmur can be caused by some type of abnormality with the heart. Examples would include holes in the walls separating chambers of the heart or abnormalities of the heart valves.

2. What is its significance?

Murmurs are only significant if they are being caused by some type of defect or abnormality with the heart. Innocent murmurs have no significance and cause no problems.

3. What are the problems that can result because of it?

The heart murmur itself does not cause any problems. However, a heart murmur that is caused by a specific heart defect will have all of the problems associated with that defect. There are numerous types of heart defects. Some are very mild and require no treatment or limitation of activity in the child. Others can be severe, requiring medication or even surgery.

4. How is it treated?

Innocent murmurs need no treatment at all. Since the heart is normal in this setting, once a murmur is determined to be innocent, no further evaluation is necessary. A heart murmur produced by an abnormality of the heart will have its treatment based on the type of abnormality that is causing the murmur.

5. What problem signs should I look for as a result of this condition?

Signs of a potential heart condition in an infant most commonly include unusual color changes (specifically a blue or pale color) or a rapid respiratory rate. In older children, heart problems can include symptoms of easy fatigue, palpitations, and, in rare cases, chest pain.

6. Is there a possibility that this condition will resolve itself without treatment?

If the heart murmur is innocent, then the heart is normal, and no further treatment or evaluation is necessary. Many innocent murmurs disappear over time, but even if an innocent murmur does not resolve, it is still not a problem. If the heart murmur is thought to be due to some type of heart defect, then the treatment will be based on the type and severity of the abnormality. Many minor heart defects require no special treatment whatsoever.

7. Will antibiotics be needed as a preventative to infection with future dental procedures?

Children with innocent heart murmurs do not require preventative antibiotics prior to dental work or surgery. In the past, antibiotics were recommended in this situation for children with actual heart defects. However, recently the American Heart Association revised their guidelines. Currently antibiotics are recommended for children with certain types of serious heart defects, for example those who have artificial heart valves or other types of prosthetic material in the heart. The vast majority of children with minor heart defects no longer require antibiotics prior to dental work or surgery.

8. Do we need to see a cardiologist?

The need to see a cardiologist is determined by your pediatrician. If your pediatrician feels comfortable that your child has an innocent murmur and the heart is normal, then no further evaluation is usually needed. If there is any concern that the murmur may not be innocent, then further evaluation by a cardiologist might be recommended.

9. When do you wish to see my child again for this condition?

Many innocent murmurs will spontaneously disappear with time as the sound qualities of the child's heart and chest change with growth. Once a heart murmur is determined to be innocent, there is no need for any further scheduled checkups with the doctor beyond the child's routine checkups. Children with heart murmurs due to heart defects need regular reevaluation, typically determined by the severity of the defect. This may be as frequently as every few months or as infrequently as once every few years.

W. PENNOCK LAIRD, II, MD
Cardiology

HEART RHYTHM IRREGULARITIES
(Arrhythmias)

Definition: Abnormal rhythm of the heartbeat.

Author's Comment: Some heart rhythm abnormalities cause no harm to the child whatsoever, while others can be life threatening. Fortunately, these are rare, but they do exist and warrant close medical scrutiny.

1. What causes this condition, and what problems does it pose for my child?

The most common type of heart rhythm abnormalities in children are due to isolated extra beats. These extra beats are termed "premature atrial contractions" if they come from the top part of the heart, or "premature ventricular contractions" if they come from the bottom. Isolated extra beats are usually benign and noticed incidentally at a routine checkup. The most common sustained arrhythmia in children is supraventricular tachycardia (SVT). This usually produces a sensation of the heart racing and can result in dizziness or, in rare cases, fainting.

2. What tests are needed to be done to better define it?

Usually an electrocardiogram (ECG) is done as a first step. More in-depth testing might include a twenty-four-hour halter monitor, which records every heartbeat for an entire day. In addition, an event monitor can be used on occasion to record the heart rhythm when a patient is having symptoms.

3. What danger signs do we need to look for?

A complaint of palpitations or a sustained, racing heart rate in a child of any age is concerning. In addition, episodes of fainting, especially related to exercise, can occasionally be caused by arrhythmias.

4. What is the treatment for this condition?

Isolated, premature atrial or ventricular contractions need no treatment whatsoever. The vast majority are benign and often resolve on their own with time. SVT generally requires treatment of some type, either medication or an invasive procedure to permanently eliminate the abnormal circuit causing the arrhythmia.

5. What precautions, if any, need to be taken in regard to limiting exercise, diet, and everyday activities?

Children with benign, isolated, premature atrial or ventricular contractions do not need any limitations whatsoever. Children diagnosed with SVT may require limitation from exercise based on the severity of the symptoms and other factors.

6. Do we need to see a cardiologist (heart specialist) and, if so, when?

Your pediatrician will decide when a referral to a cardiologist is necessary. Usually this is done if the child's symptoms are worrisome or a diagnosis of SVT has been made.

7. When do you wish to see my child again regarding this condition?

If the heart rhythm abnormality has been determined to be isolated extra beats, it is usually appropriate to reassess this on a yearly basis. Children with SVT should be checked regularly by their cardiologist, in addition to undergoing reevaluation, should they have worsening symptoms.

W. PENNOCK LAIRD, II, MD
Cardiology

HEPATITIS

Definition: Inflammation of the liver.

Author's Comment: Many cases of hepatitis contracted during childhood go undetected and get passed off frequently as some nonspecific virus because the child never becomes yellow (jaundiced). By receiving hepatitis A and B vaccines, which are given routinely in many pediatric offices, the chances of contracting this sometimes very serious disease is minimized.

1. What causes this condition, and how did my child contract it?

Hepatitis, or inflammation of the liver, can have many causes, including certain bacterial, viral, fungal, or parasitic infections. The remainder of this section will refer to the major viral causes of hepatitis: hepatitis A virus, hepatitis B virus, and hepatitis C virus.

The mode of transmission of hepatitis A virus is person-to-person via the fecal-oral route. That is, a person ingests the virus by mouth after contamination of food or a surface by the feces of an infected individual. Hepatitis B virus is transmitted from person-to-person through exposure to infected blood or certain body fluids, such as wound drainage, semen, cervical secretions, and saliva. Transmission of the hepatitis C virus can occur from person-to-person after exposure to infected blood or blood-containing fluids.

Individuals at particular risk of acquiring hepatitis B and hepatitis C include injection drug users, dialysis patients, persons who engage in high-risk sexual behavior, certain health care workers, and infants born to infected mothers. Household contacts of individuals with hepatitis B, and less so with hepatitis C, are at increased risk of acquiring the disease.

2. What diagnostic tests need to be performed to establish the cause?

The cause of hepatitis is usually established by blood testing.

3. What are the dangers or complications that are associated with this condition and are they potentially preventable?

In children, hepatitis A is usually a mild disease that occurs for a period of time and then typically goes away. In fact, many young children have no symptoms at all. Chronic infection does not occur, and complications are rare. Hepatitis A vaccine and immune globulin are effective in preventing hepatitis A. Hepatitis B and hepatitis C, on the other hand, can result in chronic infection. Over time, complications such as liver damage (cirrhosis) and liver cancer can develop. An effective vaccine is available for hepatitis B but not hepatitis C.

4. Is this condition curable, and will there be any long-term liver damage?

Hepatitis A usually resolves without specific therapy over several weeks. The risk for chronic hepatitis B infection varies greatly depending on the age at which infection occurs. For example, approximately 2 percent to 6 percent of persons infected as older children or adults will develop chronic infections, while more than 90 percent of infants infected at delivery will develop chronic disease. Up to 25 percent of individuals with chronic hepatitis B infection will develop cirrhosis or liver cancer. Approximately 50 percent to 60 percent of children with hepatitis C will develop chronic infection. Information regarding the risk of progression to cirrhosis or liver cancer in children with hepatitis C is limited, however.

5. What is the treatment?

Antiviral medications can be helpful in controlling chronic hepatitis B and hepatitis C infections in some individuals, but more effective therapies are needed.

6. Are there any specific dietary or exercise restrictions?

Under most circumstances, no dietary or exercise restrictions are necessary.

7. Is the condition contagious, and, if so, what steps need to be implemented to prevent its spread?

Children with hepatitis A, B, or C are potentially contagious, and all should be reported to the public health department. Health department officials can help assess specific situations and coordinate necessary control measures. The following discussion outlines general infection control guidelines for children with hepatitis.

Unimmunized close contacts of persons with hepatitis A, such as household members or sexual partners, should receive immune glob‐ulin. Infected children should be excluded from daycare settings until one week after the onset of the illness. Other daycare attendees and staff may require preventive therapy. Unimmunized household contacts and sexual partners of individuals with acute or chronic hepatitis B should receive the hepatitis B vaccine. Other persons who are exposed to an infected child should contact their doctor or the health department for specific recommendations. Individuals should avoid exposure to blood or possible blood‐containing body fluids of a person with hepatitis C.

8. Does any person coming into contact with my child need to receive any specific treatment or vaccination?

For more complicated situations not discussed in the previous ques‐tion, contact your doctor or the public health department for specific recommendations.

9. What signs or symptoms would warrant my calling you back?

Reasons to call include the following: confusion or difficulty awak‐ening your child, vomiting blood, and any other symptoms of concern.

10. When do you wish to see my child again regarding this condition?

Once the cause is identified, additional visits and blood tests may be necessary to assess a child's progress and determine the possible need for treatment.

STUART W. EHRETT, MD
Infectious Diseases

HERNIA (Inguinal)

Definition: A weakness in the supporting tissues of the groin area permitting the abdominal contents to bulge out.

Author's Comment: This somewhat common surgical problem can be easily repaired by a competent surgeon who deals with pediatric patients. Most children experience little discomfort following the surgery.

1. What is the cause of this condition, and how did my child develop it?

Inguinal hernias are a congenital defect in the groin muscles in children. In boys, the defect is related to the development of the testicles. The testicles actually begin development near the bottom of the kidneys during fetal development. As the fetus develops, the testicles descend and pass through the muscles of the abdomen and eventually reach the normal location on the scrotum at about six to seven months of pregnancy. If this track through the muscles (the inguinal canal) does not close properly, the "hole" in the muscles remains as a hernia. In girls, an inguinal hernia can occur through a muscular defect in which the round ligament of the uterus passes through the muscle before it inserts into the pubic bone. This defect in the muscles can be on the right side only, on the left side only, or on both sides. Though affected children are born with the hernia, it usually only becomes noticeable when the defect becomes big enough to let the intestine push through the defect and into the groin and, in boys, also the scrotum. This may occur immediately or as your child grows older. Though no one is at fault, there are several factors that can cause a hernia to develop. In small children, prematurity, asthma, and constipation can cause the hernia to develop early.

2. What are the problems that can occur as a result of this disorder?

The first problem to be encountered is called "incarceration." This occurs when intestines (or sometimes the ovary in girls) gets trapped in the hernia and will not slide back into the abdomen and cannot be pushed back in by a parent or physician. The hernia is said to be "irreducible." Symptoms may include stomachache, constipation, or vomiting, and the child may be irritable and inconsolable. Usually, if the intestines inside a hernia cannot be pushed back into the abdomen or the bulge does not go down on its own, it is considered incarcerated.

The more serious complication is called "strangulation." This usually occurs after the hernia is incarcerated. The intestine then becomes more swollen. As it swells within the hernia, the blood flow to that part of the intestine decreases, and the intestine within the hernia will eventually die, a potentially life-threatening complication. It is often apparent in boys because the groin area and scrotum are red or swollen and the child is inconsolable.

Because the hernia is visible only if intestines are pushing through the muscle, it is sometimes difficult for the surgeon to find the hernia if no intestine is "out," and a follow-up visit is all that is necessary. Sometimes the surgeon will have the family take a picture when the intestine "pokes out."

3. What are the options for treatment?

There is no medicine that will cure a congenital hernia. Treatment for congenital hernias in children is surgical repair of the hernia. This surgery is one of the most common operations performed by pediatric surgeons. In most cases it is a simple operative procedure in which the hernia is found and closed with sutures (stitches) where the hernia comes through the muscle. The surgery is well tolerated by children with minimal risk or injury. It is usually performed in an outpatient setting with most children going home that day.

The main decision in a child with only one visible hernia is how to evaluate the other side. Many studies have demonstrated that the chance that a child will have a hernia on the other side are on the order of 10 percent to 15 percent depending on the child's age. Some surgeons prefer to surgically explore the other side through another incision in the opposite groin. This option should be reserved for children with other medical problems where the possibility of a subsequent second surgical procedure should be avoided.

A second option is to not explore the other side and operate on the child later only if he or she develops a hernia on the other side. This is most acceptable in healthy children for whom the risk of another procedure later is exceedingly small.

A third option that has become more available recently is laparoscopic evaluation of the other side. In this case a small telescopic camera is passed into the abdomen through the hernia sac, and the other side is visualized from the inside. If a hernia is seen on the other side, repair of both hernias can proceed. If no hernia is seen, then the parents can be reasonably assured that a hernia will not develop on the other side. This option is being adopted by more and more pediatric surgeons.

4. What are the potential complications of surgical treatment?

Complications of hernia repair are, fortunately, quite rare. Rarely are they life threatening if recognized and managed appropriately. As in any operation, there is a small risk of bleeding or infection that may require reparation. Specific to hernias, complications include recurrence, injury to the blood supply to the testicle, and injury to the vas deferens (the tube that connects the testicle to the prostate).

5. What is the natural course if this condition is left untreated?

If untreated the hernia will do one of three things: (1) frequently, the hernia can get bigger and bigger (the author has seen a teenager where one-third of his intestine was trapped inside the scrotum); (2) incarceration; or (3) strangulation. Hernias never resolve or "fix themselves." The time progression to one of these complications may happen from days to years after the hernia first occurs with few ways to predict how quickly it will happen. However, if the hernia hurts, is persistently visible, or the child is irritable when the hernia is first noted, it is more likely to progress to incarceration or strangulation.

6. If surgery is needed, when should it occur, where, and by whom?

An appropriately trained pediatric surgeon or pediatric urologist (specialist of the urogenital tract) are the most qualified to care for children with inguinal hernias. Though older children, especially teenagers, can be cared for by adult general surgeons or urologists, the pediatric specialists typically perform more of these procedures. If the hernia is incarcerated or strangulated, the child should be taken immediately to either the surgeon's office or the emergency room for treatment. Any delay in these two conditions could result in a life-threatening complication.

7. When do you wish to see my child again for this condition?

Once a hernia is diagnosed, the surgeon will usually schedule surgery for some time within the next month. If a hernia is not seen on the first evaluation, most surgeons like to see the child again in one to two weeks for a reevaluation. X ray studies are rarely helpful and are usually of no benefit unless the surgeon thinks that there is something else causing the inguinal mass. Usually, surgeons would like to see the child two to three weeks after surgery for a postoperative visit.

KEVIN M. KADESKY, MD
Surgery

HIP JOINT INFLAMMATION (Synovitis)

Definition: An inflammation of the lining of the hip joint.

Author's Comment: This condition in childhood can cause severe pain in the hip joint when there is movement and can be an alarming symptom for the parents to observe. Fortunately, this condition resolves on its own, typically within a week, and there is no residual damage. However, other more serious causes for the hip pain need to be ruled out by your child's doctor.

1. What is the cause of this condition?

Most often, the exact cause of transient (temporary) hip joint inflammation or synovitis is unknown. The presumed cause is the result of the immune system being activated and inflamed because of an infection, such as an upper respiratory tract infection or viral infection. As a result, the immune system becomes activated, creates inflammation in the tissues, and sometimes creates inflammation in the joints, such as the hip, causing fluid and pain. This is not a true infection in the joint but inflammation of the joint. The inflammation of the joint occurs a few days to one week after the upper respiratory infection has resolved.

2. How did my child contract the inflammation?

In the same way that people get the flu, children often will develop flu-like illnesses and upper respiratory tract infections. As the immune system responds to it, the child can develop aches and pains with a transient joint inflammation or transient synovitis of the hip. It typically occurs as your body's immune system reacts to the viral infection. There is nothing one can really do to prevent this condition, not even with a vaccination.

3. What complications can develop as a result?

If this is truly transient synovitis of the hip, there are no long-term complications. This is a short-lived condition, usually lasting five to seven days, with the hip being inflamed and sore. Ultrasound or MRI can reveal extra fluid in the hip joint only. It is important to be evaluated early to have this diagnosis confirmed.

4. How long will the symptoms persist?

With transient synovitis of the hip, the limping, pain, and discomfort should last no more than seven days. Classically it will last three to five days, but up to seven days is considered okay. If the symptoms last longer than seven days, further investigation needs to be performed.

5. What tests are needed to substantiate the diagnosis? Are X rays needed?

Initially, the first part of the test is a physical examination. If the child is so sore that he or she cannot walk, then he or she needs to be seen that day at either your pediatrician's office or the emergency room to make sure it is not a bacterial joint infection that requires emergency surgery. Transient synovitis of the hip is a condition that will resolve on its own and cause no problems, but children also can develop bacterial infections in the bones and joints that present in similar fashion. If these bacterial infections are not treated very rapidly, the joint can sustain permanent damage. Therefore, it is important to confirm the diagnosis.

With transient synovitis of the hip, there is no fever. Blood work should show no signs of inflammation, meaning that the white blood cell count should be normal. Other blood tests, such as the C-reactive protein or the sedimentation rate (ESR), are markers for inflammation and should also be normal. If any of these tests are abnormal, then the concern increases about the possibility of there being infection. X rays may be needed to make certain there is not a fracture or some other condition occurring. Usually an ultrasound of the hip will show if there is fluid in the hip.

6. What is the treatment for this condition?
Before treatment, the diagnosis needs to be confirmed. Then the treatment consists of observation and the use of anti-inflammatories for a few days until the symptoms subside. The symptoms should last three to five days, but no more than seven days.

7. Is this condition contagious?
This condition is not directly contagious because it is a result of the body's immune system reacting to a viral infection. While viral infections such as the cold are contagious, developing an immune response that causes joint inflammation is dependent on the person. It is not directly contagious.

8. What activities and exercise restrictions should be imposed and for how long?

Typically for the first five to seven days while the child is having discomfort or limping, activities should be kept to a comfortable level. Walking, swimming, and bicycle riding are fine. Activities that involve a lot of jarring of the joints, such as running, jumping, or jumping on the trampoline should be avoided so as to not aggravate the joint. After one week if the child is without symptoms he or she can resume all activities.

9. Is there any need to see an orthopedist and, if so, when?

Your pediatrician is the person best trained to see initially with this problem. With his or her knowledge of you, your child, and medicine, he or she can best decide when a referral is needed. If your child is running a fever along with hip pain, has abnormal blood work, or possibly is just refusing to walk because of intense pain, an orthopedist can be useful to help manage the illness and define the cause. Infections in joints and hips can show up in the exact same manner and, if not treated within twenty-four hours, have the potential to cause permanent damage to the joint. If the child has not improved after seven days and still has limping, discomfort, or hesitation with limb movement, the child may need to be evaluated by an orthopedist, as there are other conditions that behave in a similar manner.

10. What symptoms would warrant calling the doctor again?

Symptoms lasting more than seven days, the development of a rash, development of fever, increasing limping, or other joints becoming achy, sore, of inflamed should warrant a call back to the doctor.

11. When should my child be seen again regarding this condition?

If the child's symptoms resolve in five to seven days and the child is back to normal symptomatically, there is no need for further follow-up or investigation. If the child does not follow this pattern, the child would need to return to see the doctor.

W. BARRY HUMENIUK, MD
Orthopedics

HIVES

Definition: Welt-like, sometimes blotchy, almost always itchy, red, raised eruptions on the skin.

Author's Comment: It is always alarming to see a breakout of this type on your child's skin. Most of the time the condition is not dangerous, but one is frequently left wondering as to its cause.

1. Is this a rare condition?

The medical term for hives is urticaria—a very common condition that affects approximately 20 percent to 25 percent of the population at some time in their lives. Most children have isolated cases.

2. What caused this type of eruption on my child's body to occur?

Hives are typically produced by the release of a chemical called histamine by so-called mast cells, which are found in the upper layers of the skin. Most cases of hives are classified as acute urticaria (sudden onset and relatively short lived). In this variety, the cause is more readily found. Common causes in children include: viral infection, bacterial infection (notably strep), allergic reactions to foods (especially milk, egg, peanut, fish, tree nuts, and shellfish), allergic reactions to medications including antibiotics, and allergic reactions to insect stings or bites.

Rarely, children may have chronic urticaria where hives are present on most days for six weeks or more. The cause of this condition, in many instances, is elusive.

3. Are there any serious consequences that can occur because of this condition?

Hives themselves, although uncomfortable due to itching, are harmless. They may appear on any part of the body in various different shapes and sizes and, typically, come and go. On occasion, they may be associated with angioedema—the non-itchy swelling of the deeper layers of skin, especially in soft tissue areas such as eyelids, lips, and genitals. Angioedema is due to the release of histamine in the lower skin layers. If this type of swelling occurs in areas such as the tongue or throat, it can be serious. In addition, sometimes hives may be among the first manifestations of a serious, rapid-onset, generalized allergic reaction called anaphylaxis. Anaphylaxis may include difficulty breathing, wheezing, coughing, hoarseness, difficulty swallowing, and pale, clammy skin.

4. How long do the eruptions usually last?

Hives have a tendency to come and go in crops. Characteristically, each individual hive lasts for a few minutes to several hours, but rarely for more than twenty-four to thirty-six hours. They fade without a trace. In fact, if one circles a particular hive with a marker, and it lasts for more than thirty-six hours, then the diagnosis may be in question.

New hives may tend to appear for several days or weeks, even when the cause is eliminated.

5. Are they contagious?

Hives are not contagious, although in the case where they are caused by an underlying infection (viral or bacterial), the infection itself may be contagious.

6. What tests are needed to establish the underlying cause?

A careful history and physical examination, in many instances, is all that is needed to establish a diagnosis and cause for acute urticaria. Sometimes the diagnosis may need to be confirmed with tests such as a throat culture for strep, or allergy skin tests or blood tests (such as an radioallergosorbent test or RAST) to foods or insects.

In most cases of chronic urticaria, a specific cause is not found. However, on occasion, an underlying medical condition may be the culprit. Various laboratory tests may be required to elucidate a specific diagnosis.

7. Can hives develop into a more serious condition?

Hives alone, without associated angioedema or anaphylaxis, do not develop into any serious problems.

8. What is the treatment?

If the cause or triggering factor is identifiable, eliminating exposure (where possible) may result in more rapid resolution. However, medication may still be required to help reduce the itching and clear the reaction. The initial treatment of choice is the use of prescription or nonprescription antihistamines. Benadryl and Zyrtec are available over-the-counter in all pharmacies. Alternatively, nonsedating antihistamines such as Claritin or Alavert are also available over-the-counter. More difficult cases are often treated with combinations of antihistamines and/or addition of histamine H2 blockers such as Zantac or Tagamet. Stronger treatments are available for more resistant cases.

It is best to temporarily avoid overheating as well as the use of aspirin, Advil, or Motrin, and Aleve, as these may intensify or prolong the hive episode. Cool baths or applications of cool compresses may be helpful to reduce itching and swelling. However, application of Benadryl cream or cortisone-based creams is not typically beneficial. Administering antihistamines regularly until the rash is clear for twenty-four to forty-eight hours is advisable.

9. Are there any side effects from the treatment?

Older antihistamines such as Benadryl and Atarax can cause drowsiness in some children. Xyzal, a prescription antihistamine, and Zyrtec may also cause drowsiness, but this is rare. Claritin or Alavert as well as the prescription products Allegra and Clarinex, do not cause sedation.

10. Do we need to see an allergist or dermatologist?

An allergist should be consulted in cases where acute urticaria does not have an obvious or previously defined trigger; when acute urticaria is caused by a presumed food, drug, or insect allergy with the need for diagnostic confirmation or assistance with avoidance; as well as in cases of chronic urticaria. A dermatologist should be consulted if the individual welts consistently last for more than thirty-six hours and, especially, if they leave residual purple or otherwise discolored skin.

11. When should I call you back?

You should call back

- immediately, if there are signs of anaphylaxis (including wheezing, throat tightness, shortness of breath, hoarseness, etc.);
- immediately, if your child has a history of severe allergy to food or insect sting and is definitely exposed;
- if your child is uncomfortable with little to no relief with over-the-counter or prescribed antihistamines;
- if your child has any adverse affects from the medications;
- if your child looks very ill; or
- if you are concerned and/or have additional questions.

12. When do you want to see my child again regarding this condition?

Your child should be seen again, if

- the hives become more severe or persist in spite of the regular dosing of antihistamines;
- most of the itching is not relieved with the continuous use of antihistamines, interfering with school and normal activities;
- your child becomes worse or develops swelling of the lips, eyelids, tongue, or other areas;
- your child develops fever, abdominal pain, and swollen joints;
- you are concerned and think your child needs to be seen.

ELLIOT J. GINCHANSKY, MD
Allergy and Immunology

HYDROCELE (of the Testes)

Definition: **Fluid in the scrotum surrounding the testicle.**

Author's Comment: This condition, which frequently occurs at birth, can either resolve on its own or require surgical intervention and repair. Your child's doctor will be able to differentiate which type of hydrocele it is and whether your child will need to see a surgeon.

1. What is the cause of this condition, and how did it develop in my child?

Hydroceles in newborns are the result of fluid trapped around the testicle that results when the testicle descends into the scrotum in the fetus. There are two types:

- **Congenital hydrocele:** Fluid is trapped around the testicle when the passageway to the scrotum (inguinal canal) closes. This fluid can vary in size but typically will resolve before the child reaches a year of age. A hydrocele of the cord is a variation of the congenital hydrocele, in which the fluid is not in the scrotum but in the inguinal canal.

- **Communicating hydrocele:** In these cases, a small connection occurs between the hydrocele and the abdominal cavity. As a result, the hydrocele will vary in size throughout the day (usually smaller in the morning and bigger at night).

Hydroceles that occur rapidly in older children may be the result of other underlying serious problems including testicular torsion, epididymitis, orchitis, trauma, and, rarely, testicular tumors. These typically occur in older children and often have other symptoms like fever, pain, localized redness, or sudden onset.

2. What are the problems that can occur as a result of this disorder?

Usually the most important concern with a hydrocele is to differentiate it from an incarcerated hernia. Normally, this can be done by direct examination by the child's pediatrician or family doctor. If of concern, pediatric surgeons and pediatric urologists can frequently make the diagnosis. Hydroceles more frequently have a bluish discoloration and do not cause any discomfort. Rarely, studies like an ultrasound need to be performed to differentiate the two.

Newborn congenital hydroceles rarely cause problems. Communicating hydroceles tend to get bigger with time but will not cause any true symptoms until they get quite large. Any serious problems are caused by unrecognized conditions that cause a secondary hydrocele, though these cases usually have other symptoms or an unusual history.

3. What are the options for treatment?

Treatment for congenital hydroceles in children is surgical repair of the hydrocele. There is no medicine that will cure a congenital hydrocele. In most cases, the hydrocele is found and resected (open widely) in a simple operation. Sometimes, the connection with the abdominal cavity needs to be found and tied off. The surgery is well tolerated by children with minimal risk or injury. It is usually performed in an outpatient setting with most children going home that day.

4. What are the potential complications of surgical treatment?

Complications of hydrocele repair are, fortunately, quite rare. Rarely are they life threatening if recognized and managed appropriately. As in any operation, there is a small risk of bleeding or infection that may require reparation. Specific to hernias, complications include recurrence, injury to the blood supply to the testicle, and injury to the vas deferens (the tube that connects the testicle to the prostate).

5. What is the natural course if the condition is left untreated?

If untreated, the hydrocele will do one of three things:

- It will get bigger and bigger.
- It will remain the same size.
- It will resolve on its own. This is the most common course for newborns with hydroceles.

6. If surgery is needed, when should it occur, where, and by whom?

An appropriately trained pediatric urologist or pediatric surgeon are the most qualified to care for children with congenital hydroceles.

Though older children, especially teenagers, can be cared for by adult general surgeons or urologists, the pediatric specialists typically perform more of these procedures. Repair of a persistent congenital hydrocele or communicating hydrocele can be scheduled electively at the family's convenience.

7. When do you wish to see my child again for this condition?

A surgeon will typically want to see a newborn with a congenital hydrocele at about one year old. If the hydrocele is still present, surgery may be required to repair the hydrocele. After surgery, most surgeons will want to see the child for a visit at two to three weeks after surgery.

KEVIN M. KADESKY, MD
Surgery

HYPERTENSION

Definition: **High blood pressure.**

Author's Comment: High blood pressure, though rare, is always a worrisome finding in children and should be evaluated for an underlying cause before beginning a treatment plan. A blood pressure reading should always be a routine part of your child's yearly physical exam.
Note: A blood pressure cuff that is too small for a larger arm (often seen during adolescence) can give an artificially high blood pressure reading.

1. What causes this condition?
There are two main categories for hypertension. The first is primary or essential hypertension, which has no identifiable cause. Children with primary hypertension are frequently overweight. Data obtained from school health-screening programs demonstrate that the prevalence of hypertension increases progressively with increasing body mass index, and there is a strong association of hypertension with obesity. Environmental conditions can also affect blood pressure. This includes time of day, ambient temperature, seasonal variability,

activity, and mood. There is a strong genetic influence on blood pressure. Children from families with a history of hypertension are at a higher risk as compared to children without any notable family history. Race is also considered a factor in the development of elevated blood pressure. The prevalence of hypertension is greater in blacks as compared to whites. Data from other ethnic groups are not currently available.

The next category is secondary hypertension. This is more common in children than in adults. The possibility that some underlying disorder may be the cause of hypertension should be considered in every child. The most common underlying cause of secondary hypertension is renal or kidney disease. Another cause of secondary hypertension is a congenital narrowing or constriction of a large artery arising from the heart called the aorta. This condition, called "coarctation of the aorta," creates a situation where the blood pressure in the arms is higher than the blood pressure in the legs. Other less common causes of secondary hypertension include tumors or disorders of the adrenal gland and the use of certain medications, such as oral contraceptives, steroids, antihistamines, decongestants, and nutritional supplements aimed at enhancing athletic performance.

2. What potential problems can it lead to, and what are the long-term effects of this condition?

High blood pressure in childhood has been considered a risk factor for hypertension in early adulthood. Hypertension is a risk factor for cardiovascular disease, stroke, and damage to organs affected by the elevated blood pressure (end-organ damage). The most prominent evidence of end-organ damage is thickening of the left lower pumping chamber of the heart or left ventricle. Other examples of end-organ damage include scarring of the kidneys, thickening of the carotid or coronary arteries and changes in the arteries of the retina. Elevated blood pressure is also associated with other problems such as elevated cholesterol, diabetes mellitus, and sleep disorders.

3. What tests are needed to better understand why this condition occurred?

Several tests can be helpful in the evaluation of hypertension. Blood chemistry levels and urinalysis may be able to identify an underlying disorder in the kidneys. A renal ultrasound can identify any structural abnormality of the kidneys. An echocardiogram is an ultrasound of the heart that can rule out constriction of the aorta and evaluate the thickness of the left ventricle. A drug screen may help identify certain substances that can lead to hypertension. Other tests such as CT scan, magnetic resonance angiography (MRA), or arteriography can help in identifying any narrowing of the arterial or venous system of the kidneys that can lead to hypertension.

4. Is hypertension curable?

In many children, therapeutic lifestyle changes and pharmacologic (drug) therapy, if needed, are often curative in the treatment of essential hypertension. Other children will continue to require therapy.

5. What medicines are used to treat this disorder, and what can we hope to accomplish with this treatment?

Indications for drug therapy include secondary hypertension, and the presence of clinical symptoms, such as chronic headaches, dizziness, lethargy, established damage to bodily organs, and a lack of response to lifestyle modifications. Pharmacologic therapy should be initiated with a single drug. There are approximately nine different classes of drugs and numerous drugs in each class or category to choose from. All classes of antihypertensive drugs have been shown to be effective in lowering blood pressure in children and, therefore, the choice for initial therapy resides in the preference of your child's physician. Some of the more common classes of medications that are prescribed include beta-blockers and diuretics. However, recently some of the newer classes of antihypertensive drugs, such as angiotensin-converting enzyme inhibitors (ACE) are easier to dose and have fewer side effects. The goal of any antihypertensive therapy in children is reduction of the blood pressure to less than the 95th percentile, based on normative values for weight and height.

6. What are the side effects of the medicines?

Side effects of the medications depend on the specific drug. For example, use of diuretics lead to increased frequency of urination, which can cause low potassium levels. Therefore, these drugs are usually used in conjugation with potassium supplements. Other less common side effects of diuretics include glucose intolerance and elevation of serum lipid levels. Beta-blockers can lead to worsening respiratory symptoms in patients with underlying asthma or related conditions. These drugs also lower the heart rate and can impair athletic performance or cause lethargy. ACE inhibitors are not given in pregnancy because of known adverse effects on the fetus.

7. Are there any other ways to control the blood pressure?

Weight reduction is the primary therapy for obesity-related hypertension. Regular physical activity and restriction of sedentary activity are also important in the prevention of obesity and helps prevent an excess increase in blood pressure over time. Dietary modification should be in the form of smaller-sized portions, a decrease in the consumption of sugar-containing beverages and energy-dense snacks, and an increase in consumption of fresh fruits and vegetables, nonfat dairy, and regular meals including breakfast. Foods rich in fiber have been shown to be beneficial as well. Sodium reduction is essential in the management of hypertension. Recent data have also shown that calcium supplementation and increased intake of potassium, magnesium, and folic acid is associated with lower blood pressure.

8. What restrictions in diet, exercise, and daily activities need to be imposed?

In addition to the recommendations discussed in question #7, smoking and excessive alcohol intake should be avoided. Parents should monitor how much time a child spends in sedentary activities such as watching television and playing video games. These activities should be limited to less than two hours daily. Regular aerobic activity of thirty to sixty minutes three to four times weekly should be encouraged. Power weightlifting is not advised, but resistance training can be helpful. Competitive sports are also not advised in children or adolescents with a blood pressure consistently more than 5 mmHg above the 99th percentile, based on normative values for weight and height.

9. Are there any danger signs that we need to look for that might indicate a complication of this disorder?

Frequent headaches, dizziness, and vision changes are some clinical manifestations of hypertension. Changes in the urine such as dark urine or blood in the urine could point toward a kidney related cause for the hypertension. Chest pain, shortness of breath, or palpitations in an older child or adolescent might be a sign of a cardiac complication. Seizures, vomiting, or a decreased level of consciousness require prompt or emergency evaluation.

10. Should we consult a specialist in this type of disorder and, if so, when?

Pediatric subspecialists can play an important role along with your child's pediatrician in the management of hypertension. A nutritionist can be helpful in dietary modification or suggestions and can provide customized recommendations. A pediatric nephrologist (kidney specialist) can recommend specific tests that can unveil an underlying cause and be extremely helpful in drug management, especially if multiple medications are needed. A pediatric cardiologist can provide routine echocardiograms to evaluate for end-organ damage, such as monitoring the thickness of the left ventricle and to rule out coarctation of the aorta, which is one of the major secondary causes of hypertension. A cardiologist can also be helpful in pharmacological management of hypertension.

11. When do you wish to see my child again regarding the high blood pressure?

Any child with hypertension should have his or her blood pressure monitored regularly. Home (stationary) or ambulatory (walking) blood pressure monitoring is helpful to aid in monitoring a patient in different settings, at different times of day. Any patient with an elevated blood pressure or a patient on medications should have his or her blood pressure monitored several times weekly. An elevated blood pressure must be confirmed on repeated visits before a child is characterized as having hypertension, usually multiple readings taken over weeks to months. Once a patient has been labeled as having hypertension, visits to the physician should occur no less than twice yearly. If medical management is initiated, more frequent visits at the onset are needed to evaluate response and/or side effects.

JANE KAO, MD
Cardiology

HYPOTHYROIDISM

Definition: **Low-functioning thyroid.**

Author's Comment: The thyroid gland is one of the prime regulators of metabolic function in the body. A low-functioning thyroid gland therefore affects the body in many negative ways.

1. What are the major bodily symptoms of hypothyroidism?

The symptoms associated with hypothyroidism depend upon the age of the child with the disorder. In newborns, there are very few symptoms, but after a few months, untreated hypothyroidism will show itself with symptoms of failure to thrive, poor alertness, sallow skin, and lack of achievement of developmental milestones.

In older children, the symptoms are those which one might expect with a slow down in metabolism—they may include constipation, slow growth, fatigue, dry hair and dry skin, hair loss, a feeling of being colder than others around them, and pallor. Interestingly, children with hypothyroidism do not tend to be obese. Because their metabolic rate is lowered, they are not as hungry as normal and tend to gain weight slowly.

2. What caused this condition to occur in my child?

One in four thousand infants is born with an absent or poorly functioning thyroid gland. The exact causes of this are currently unknown.
In older children, hypothyroidism is generally caused when the
immune system attacks the thyroid gland and reduces its function.

3. What tests need to be done to evaluate this disorder?

A visit with the pediatrician is very important so that any symptoms
associated with hypothyroidism can be noted. A physical exam is also
very important to check for a possible goiter, or enlargement of the
thyroid gland, or signs of pallor, dry skin, or poor growth. A suggestive
history and physical will allow the pediatrician to decide if blood tests
need to be done. These blood tests may include a direct measure of the
thyroid hormones, thyroxine (T4), and triiodothyronine (T3), a
measure of the brain hormone that regulates thyroid hormone production (TSH), or a measure of antibodies to the thyroid gland.

4. What is the treatment for this condition, and are there any major side effects that can occur as a result of the treatment?

The treatment of this condition is with oral administration of thyroid
hormone replacement. The most widely used product is identical to
the T4 that the human thyroid gland makes normally. T4 is normally
converted to T3 in the body, and therefore it is frequently not necessary to also give T3.

Since the products used currently are identical to the thyroid
hormone that the normal gland makes, the side effects of the replacement therapy are minimal and dose related. If a child's dose is too low,

his or her symptoms will not go away. If the dose is too high, difficulty sleeping, nervousness, sweatiness, and heart palpitations may occur.

In newborns that are diagnosed with congenital hypothyroidism, prompt treatment is crucial to preserve cognitive ability. The risks of not treating this disorder in babies are far more severe than any minimal risk of the medication.

5. Can my child lead a normal life with appropriate treatment?

Yes. Although treatment involves taking a medication daily and periodic visits to the doctor with lab tests, most children do not view themselves as "sick," and medication and doctor visits become routine to them.

6. Do we need to consult with a pediatric endocrinologist for this disorder?

Pediatric endocrinologists are pediatricians who have spent several extra years in training to learn about hormone disorders in children. Therefore, they are a valuable resource to you and your pediatrician. Most babies with congenital hypothyroidism are followed very closely by both the pediatric endocrinologist and the pediatrician. Many older children also find the assistance of a pediatric endocrinologist valuable.

7. What kind of follow-up will be needed in the future?

As a child grows, thyroid hormone requirements can change. Therefore, during periods of rapid growth, such as infancy, frequent visits with lab testing will be needed in order to optimally replace thyroid hormone. As a child grows, visits can range from every four to six months to once a year. Obviously, the schedule of follow-up will need to be tailored to the individual's needs.

ELLEN S. SHER, MD
Endocrinology

INGROWN TOENAIL

Definition: A condition where the toenail grows into the flesh of the surrounding skin.

Author's Comment: This condition is an argument for good fitting shoes and for cutting toenails straight across as opposed to on a curve.

1. What causes this condition?

An ingrown toenail occurs when a corner or side of the nail curves down into the skin. It can also occur if there is a "hangnail" or a split nail. The most common causes for an ingrown toenail to occur are improperly (tightly) fitting shoes and improper cutting of the nail. Other causes can include trauma, such as being stepped on while playing sports, cutting the nails with instruments not meant for that purpose, such as a paper scissor, or even picking at a toenail with your fingers because the nail is too long.

2. What is the treatment?

If there is mild discomfort, treatment can be as simple as soaking the foot in warm water with Epsom Salts or Domeboro Soaks. Wear an open-toe or wide-toe shoe to avoid pressure on the nail. Use a cuticle stick to lift the corner of the nail up and out of the skin. Caution: do not push the cuticle too far under the nail, just the loose corner.

If there is discomfort where the mildest of pressure causes discomfort, such as a bed sheet or even putting your sock and/or shoe on or if there appears to be an infection, then you should see your doctor. Treatment for an ingrown nail with an infection might be as simple as using foot soaks with a prescription for a topical and/or oral antibiotic.

If the infection or pain is severe enough, then surgical removal of the nail border is performed. Depending on the severity of the infection your doctor may prescribe an oral antibiotic.

3. If surgery is needed, will it be painful?

The injection of the local anesthetic to the toe might result in a burning sensation, but it is a momentary discomfort. Once the toe is numb there should be no discomfort during the procedure. When the toe wakes up there might be a tingling sensation. If there is discomfort, then an over-the-counter pain reliever (acetaminophen or ibuprofen) would be appropriate.

4. Can there be complications from surgical treatment?

The most common, although not frequent, complications could include discomfort, continued pain, continued infection, swelling, and/or recurrence. If the infected toe is not treated, the complication can be more serious and could lead to a bone infection.

5. Do we need to see an orthopedist (bone specialist) or a podiatrist (foot specialist)?

Your pediatrician will decide when and if a referral is necessary. Some pediatricians feel comfortable treating simple ingrown toenails with or without infection. For more complicated or recurrent ingrown toenails, a referral is usually indicated to a foot or bone specialist who is more accustomed to treating this type of disorder.

6. What can we do to prevent recurrence of this condition?

The following can be done in an attempt to prevent recurrence, but sometimes an ingrown nail just occurs again. Prevention can include the following:

- Wear properly fitting socks and shoes.
- If there is trauma to the toe or nail, inspect it. If it appears that the nail is damaged or there is discomfort, start soaks.
- Properly trim the nails, using appropriate toenail-trimming tools. Do not cut the toenail too short, and cut the nail straight across (if you have a sharp corner, use a nail file to round the corner).

7. When do you wish to see my child again?

Following surgical removal of the ingrown nail border, there is a follow-up visit approximately ten days after the procedure. If there are questions or abnormal postsurgical discomfort, then seeing the patient sooner would be appropriate.

DONALD BLUM, DPM
Podiatry

INSECT BITE

Definition: A bite on the skin caused by an insect.

Author's Comment: Treating symptoms alone is usually enough for most of these occurrences, unless you suspect that the bite came from a poisonous critter. If so, consult with your child's doctor.

1. What can be done to lessen the symptoms caused from this bite?

Itching may be relieved by calamine lotion, but avoid application on the areas around the eyes and genitals. Holding a cloth soaked in cold water over the area may lessen discomfort. Acetaminophen or ibuprofen may also be helpful.

2. Is there anything needed to prevent the area from getting infected?

Wash the wound well with soap and water, and then keep the area clean and dry. Also, make sure your child's tetanus immunizations are up to date.

3. If this is a spider bite, how do we know it is not a toxic spider bite?

The brown recluse spider and the black widow spider are the two most dangerous spiders in North America. If the spider is available and can be captured safely, take it to your physician for identification. If the spider is not available, observe closely and call if the area becomes painful, blistered, or discolored; if muscle spasms occur; or if your child seems especially ill. Bites from other spiders may cause less serious, local reactions.

4. If this is a tick bite, how do we know that the bite is not from the type of tick that causes Lyme disease?

Lyme disease can be transmitted by more than one species of tick, and the ticks capable of carrying the Lyme disease bacteria (*Borrelia burgdorferi*) vary between geographical regions. If the tick is still attached, remove it as soon as possible. The most widely recommended method of tick removal is to use a tweezers and grasp the tick carefully as close to the skin surface as possible. Then pull upward gently until the tick is removed and wash the area well with soap and water. If part of the tick remains embedded, call your doctor. If the tick is available, take it to your doctor, who can either identify it or send it to a specialist who can. Preventive medication is not usually necessary.

5. What signs or developments would warrant our getting back in touch with you?

After a bite or sting, reasons to call back include fever, headache, muscle pain or spasms, skin rashes, significant redness, discoloration, swelling or pain at the site, difficulty breathing, unusual sensations, or any symptoms of concern.

6. What kind of follow-up is needed?

No follow-up is usually needed unless you notice any of the symptoms discussed earlier.

STUART W. EHRETT, MD

Infectious Diseases

ITP
(Idiopathic Thrombocytopenia Purpura)

Definition: Small hemorrhages into the skin due to the deficiency of one of the blood clotting elements, not connected with any definable disease.

Author's Comment: If you see little purple flat spots appear all over the body, they may represent small hemorrhages (petechiae) in the skin and warrant having your child seen by the doctor immediately.

1. What causes this condition, and how did my child contract it?

ITP is due to a mistake made by the child's immune system. When a child develops an infection, the child fights the infection with the immune system. The immune system consists of several parts, including certain white blood cells and certain proteins in the body called antibodies. Certain white blood cells in the body called lymphocytes make antibodies. Antibodies then attack the germ, whether it be a virus or a bacteria. Sometimes, by mistake, the antibodies also attack the child's own platelets. When this happens, the body thinks that the platelets must be germs, and the antibody-coated platelets are removed from the child's circulation. This causes a very low platelet count and causes the child to bruise easily and also may cause nosebleeds or blood in the urine or stool. The problems with bleeding and low platelet count generally occur after the infection has already resolved. In most cases, children with ITP look otherwise healthy except for the bleeding problems.

2. How long will it last, and is it completely curable?

About 80 percent of children with ITP will completely recover within six months. For most children, there is never a recurrence of the disorder. In approximately 20 percent of children with ITP, the problem may last longer than six months and may recur in the future. However, many of these patients will eventually be completely cured as well.

3. What are the complications of this disorder?

Most children with ITP will have unexplained bruises over many parts of the body. Some children will also have problems with nosebleeds or possibly blood in the urine or stool. Severe, life-threatening bleeding is quite unusual and occurs probably in less than one in a hundred children with this disorder. The most serious complication would be internal bleeding such as bleeding in the brain. However, again, it should be emphasized that this is not common.

4. Do we need to see a hematologist (a specialist in blood disorders), and does my child need to be hospitalized?

Some pediatricians are perfectly comfortable at treating a child with ITP. On occasion, a pediatric hematology consultation is requested. Depending upon the amount of bleeding, and the level of the platelet count, the child might need to be hospitalized. However, the majority of children with ITP do not need to be in the hospital.

5. What is the treatment for this disorder, and are there any potential side effects?

The majority of patients with ITP will recover without treatment. Pediatricians and pediatric hematologists do not all agree on which patients should be treated. There are medications that can speed up the recovery of the platelet count. Although the medications are generally well tolerated, sometimes they can have bothersome side effects and can be very expensive. Many pediatric hematologists will recommend treatment for young children with ITP who have very low platelet counts (below 10,000) and who exhibit signs of bleeding anywhere other than the skin. So, for example, a three-year-old child with a platelet count of 2,000 who has been having nosebleeds is more likely to receive treatment than a twelve-year-old child with a platelet count of 25,000 who is only exhibiting bleeding in the skin. The decision to treat is generally made with the input of the pediatrician, the pediatric hematologist, and the family.

6. What kind of exercise limitations need to be imposed, and when will my child be able to resume a normal routine?

In general, a physician will recommend no contact sports and reduced physical activity when the platelet count is low. The child will be able to resume a normal routine when the platelet count has returned to a normal level. A normal level usually means a platelet count greater than 100,000, although some patients with platelet count between 50,000 and 100,000 can also resume normal activities.

7. How often do we need to have follow-up blood tests?

A child will generally need to have blood tests performed several times in the first six months after diagnosis. Further blood tests will depend upon the needs of the individual child.

8. When do you wish to see my child again for this disorder?

Children with ITP are generally seen several times in the first month after diagnosis. Follow-up exams will depend upon the child's speed of recovery or response to treatment.

CARL LENARSKY, MD

Hematology

KIDNEY INFECTION
(Pyelonephritis)

Definition: Infection of the kidneys.

Author's Comment: This condition needs to be treated aggressively to totally eradicate the infection. It is of the utmost importance that you follow up with your child's doctor. Further testing may be necessary to rule out any underlying structural abnormalities that could possibly lead to recurrent infections.

1. What is the cause of this condition, and how did my child contract it?

Pyelonephritis occurs when an infectious agent gains access to the kidney and begins to multiply. Most kidney infections start off as infections in the bladder and ascend up into the kidneys. In some children, especially in newborns, pyelonephritis can occur due to bacteria traveling through the bloodstream and reaching the kidney through blood vessels. Most of the bacteria that cause pyelonephritis can be found in the stool. The most common cause of pyelonephritis is a bacteria called *E. coli*.

2. What complications can occur as a result of this condition?

Complications include development of high blood pressure (hypertension), kidney scarring, kidney abscess formation (collection of pus in the kidney), and kidney failure. Prompt diagnosis, treatment, and prevention of future episodes will decrease the likelihood of these complications.

3. What is the treatment?

Antibiotics are the mainstay of treatment for children with pyelonephritis. Very young children with this condition, or children of any age with severe nausea, vomiting, or dehydration, may require admission to the hospital for inpatient treatment with intravenous antibiotics and fluid administration. Studies have shown that certain kinds of oral antibiotics are just as effective as intravenous antibiotics for treatment of pyelonephritis. The length of prescribed treatment may vary from seven to fourteen days.

4. What are the potential side effects of the treatment?

Many different types of antibiotics can be used to treat pyelonephritis. Ideally, antibiotic selection should be tailored to the specific sensitivities of the bacteria causing your child's infection. Each type of antibiotic has certain side effects that your physician can discuss with you. The most commonly seen side effects are upset stomach, skin rashes, diarrhea, or yeast infections.

5. What diagnostic tests should be performed to determine any underlying structural cause?

Children of any age that develop pyelonephritis should be evaluated with an ultrasound of the kidneys and bladder and a bladder test called a voiding cystourethrogram (VCUG). The ultrasound can reveal any structural anomalies of the kidneys, ureter, or bladder that may predispose to pyelonephritis. The bladder test (VCUG) will evaluate for vesicoureteral reflux (urine washing back up into the kidneys), bladder abnormalities, and problems with the urinary channel to the skin (the urethra). Additionally, there are certain circumstances when your physician may wish to obtain a nuclear medicine test called a DMSA renal scan. This can confirm the diagnosis of pyelonephritis in the acute phase (when the child is severly ill) and look for evidence of kidney scarring in the long term.

6. Do we need to see a urologist?

A urologist should be involved if there are any structural or functional problems detected during the evaluation. Also, patients with recurrent episodes of pyelonephritis with a normal evaluation may benefit from seeing a urologist.

7. Will there be any physical restrictions placed on my child because of this condition?

Typically there are no restrictions recommended for patients with pyelonephritis pending their evaluation.

8. What symptoms would prompt me to call you back again?

It is not uncommon for children to continue to have elevated temperatures for a few days after starting antibiotic treatment. This can be seen especially at night. However, if your child has persistent fever beyond this period, your physician may wish to repeat urinary studies or change the antibiotic regimen to broaden the coverage.

Consideration may also be given to obtaining a CT scan to look for a kidney abscess. Blood in the urine, worsening back or abdominal pain, or persistence of other symptoms are reasons to notify your physician.

9. What kind of follow-up will be needed to make sure this infection has been eradicated?

A repeat urine culture obtained one to two weeks after completion of the antibiotic course can be useful to make sure the infection has been eradicated. Some physicians will want to make sure that there is no evidence of residual infection before the bladder X rays are performed.

WILLIAM STRAND, MD
Urology

LARGE HEAD
(Macrocephaly)

Author's Comment: When the doctor measures your infant's head each time you come in for a checkup, it is to make sure that the child's head is growing at a normal rate. A large head can represent a significant problem in the structure of the growing brain. Some children, however, just have big heads with no underlying problems.

1. What caused this condition to occur in my child?

Macrocephaly is defined as the head size being more than two standard deviations above the average. This is normal in approximately 5 percent of children. However, this can also be a sign of a problem with the brain or the bones of the skull. If there is a problem it could be from the accumulation of too much cerebrospinal fluid in the skull (hydrocephalus). In addition, a very large head could be an indication of abnormal brain formation, a metabolic defect, genetic problems, or bone problems as in achondroplasia (abnormal conversion of cartilage into bone).

2. What future implications does it pose as to my child's learning and intellectual function?

Future implications depend on the causes. Some children will have cognitive defects, attention difficulties, movement disorders, or epilepsy.

3. What diagnostic tests are needed to further establish the cause and define the condition?

Depending on the history and physical examination, tests such as an MRI of the brain, genetic or metabolic testing as well as an electroencephalogram (EEG) may be useful.

4. Does it represent any underlying problem with the structure of the brain or could it be part of a more generalized condition?

The cause for macrocephaly, if known, can tell us if the problem is just the brain or if there is a more generalized problem.

5. What is the proposed treatment for this condition, and how successful is it?

If the cause for the macrocephaly is hydrocephalus, treatment could include a shunt to drain excess cerebrospinal fluid from the brain into the abdominal cavity, or other surgery for hydrocephalus. Some metabolic treatments may also be available if the macrocephaly is caused by a metabolic disorder. Treatment is based on what other problems the child has such as epilepsy.

6. Is there a specialist that we should consult and, if so, when?

Various specialists can help when this condition becomes apparent. They include a pediatric neurologist, pediatric neurosurgeon, geneticist, physical medicine and rehabilitation specialist, or developmental pediatrician.

7. Are there any genetic factors associated with this condition?

Yes, some cases of macrocephaly are genetic in origin.

8. When do you wish to see my child again regarding this condition?

Follow-up with the pediatrician depends on what other problems the child has and how severe they are.

DAVID B. OWEN, MD
Neurology

LARYNGITIS

Definition: **Inflammation of the larynx.**

Author's Comment: Hoarseness is usually the most prominent symptom of this condition. One goal of the treatment plan should be to rest the voice. Most children, however, will have no part of this. You may have to rely on a good humidifier, exercise restrictions, and possibly some prescription medicines to recover.

1. What causes this condition to occur, and how did my child contract it?

Laryngitis is an inflammation of the voice box (larynx). The inflammation results in redness and mild edema (swelling of the vocal cords and adjacent structures). Hoarseness is usually the most prominent symptom of this condition. Laryngitis is often associated with an upper respiratory tract infection (a cold). The infection is usually viral and may be associated with clear nasal drainage and cough. A child with allergic nasal symptoms may develop laryngitis associated with an acute flare-up of the allergy symptoms. Occasionally, bacteria cause not only laryngitis but other more significant symptoms. The child may be acutely ill with fever and a significant cough. Since most of the acute cases of laryngitis are infectious, the child contracts the illness from another person.

2. Is it contagious, and how is it spread?

Viral and bacterial infections are contagious and are usually spread by microdroplets from other individuals through contact, cough, or sneezing.

3. What complications can possibly occur as a result of this disorder?

Acute laryngitis lasts from three to five days. Resolution of the hoarseness or vocal changes is accompanied by improvement in the child's cough and other respiratory symptoms such as nasal congestion and drainage. Prolonged laryngitis is indicative of a more chronic condition of the larynx with possible changes of the lining of the vocal cord. These changes may simply be prolonged redness and swelling of focal (localized) areas of vocal cord thickening, such as a vocal cord nodule. Focal inflammation can also be the result of a condition called a granuloma.

4. How is it treated?

Acute laryngitis is a self-limited problem; it occurs for a period of time, and then typically goes away. If it is a result of a viral infection and associated with clear nasal drainage and cough, treatment consists of increased humidity such as a cool mist humidifier, voice rest (if possible in a child), increased hydration, and possible use of pain medications such as acetaminophen or ibuprofen.

Antibiotics have not been shown to be beneficial unless the child is acutely ill with fever and other symptoms such as a significant "barking cough" consistent with a problem called acute laryngotracheobronchitis. This inflammatory problem not only involves the vocal cords but also the trachea (windpipe) and bronchi (large airways of the lungs). More aggressive treatment with antibiotics, humidification, and possibly steroids may be used.

Laryngitis that lasts for longer than two weeks needs to be evaluated to determine if the child has chronic inflammation of the larynx. Examination of the larynx is performed by way of visual inspection through laryngoscopy. Provided the child is cooperative, this may be accomplished in the office with a flexible, fiber optic laryngoscope that records video. Occasionally, a child needs to undergo general anesthesia for inspection of the larynx. If the laryngoscopy reveals marked swelling and redness, then steroids are occasionally used on a short-term basis—less than one week. Mild-to-moderate edema in a child with persistent symptoms of hoarseness may indicate reflux of stomach acid to the level of the larynx. This condition is treated with a medication to decrease stomach acid production. The antireflux medication most commonly given to children is Prilosec or Prevacid on a twice-daily basis.

Allergy medications, such as antihistamines and steroid sprays, are used in those children with laryngitis and allergic symptoms.

Focal areas of inflammation, such as granulomas, are treated surgically by laryngoscopy and removal. However, chronic hoarseness is best treated conservatively with speech therapy.

5. If medicines are to be used, what side effects can occur?

As mentioned, acute laryngitis is treated conservatively without antibiotics and steroids. Medications for reflux, such as Prevacid or

Prilosec, are very well tolerated. Occasionally, children complain of abdominal pain and diarrhea with these medications. The newer antihistamines used in allergic children have minimal side effects of drowsiness and dryness of the nasal lining.

6. How long will it take for my child to show improvement?

Most children with acute viral laryngitis get better within three to five days with conservative therapy. However, for those with acute bacterial laryngotracheal bronchitis, the hoarseness and cough may last for one to two weeks.

Most children with reflux require treatment for at least two months before definite improvement in vocal quality is noted. Those children diagnosed with the vocal cord nodules require an extended period of time of speech therapy to alter vocal patterns that result in injury of the lining and thickening of the vocal cord.

Control of the inhalant allergies with improvement in nasal congestion usually accompanies the improvement in the laryngitis and vocal quality.

7. When can my child return to school and resume physical activities?

Children with acute laryngitis improve their vocal quality as the symptoms of upper respiratory tract infection resolve, including resolution of the cough, nasal drainage, and fever. When these symptoms have improved, the child may resume physical activities.

Those children that experience vocal cord nodules may be restricted in activities that would result in vocal overuse such as screaming and shouting.

8. Will my child now be more prone to developing laryngitis on a recurrent basis?

Recurrent laryngitis is usually related to two factors. First, reflux can occur on an intermittent basis, causing inflammation and hoarseness after initial treatment is discontinued. If this is the case, then a decision between the physician and the parent will need to be made as to the continuation of reflux medications on a continual basis.

Second, vocal overuse or misuse can result in vocal inflammation and vocal cord thickening, requiring continued vocal therapy. A speech pathologist generally follows these children over an extended period of time to ensure good vocal hygiene and voice patterns.

9. What signs do we look for to make sure the condition is not getting worse?

Changes in the vocal quality of the voice, most notably noisy breathing (airway noise), possibly indicate worsening of the condition, warranting further clinical investigation.

10. When do you wish to see my child again for follow-up?

Acute laryngitis is a self-limited problem that usually goes away in seven to ten days. If your child continues to experience changes in vocal quality, then a reassessment will need to occur within two to three weeks.

In children that experience chronic laryngitis and are being treated either for vocal inflammation (vocal cord nodule or granuloma) or reflux, a reassessment will need to occur in two to three months.

TIMOTHY TRONE, MD
Otolaryngology

LEARNING DIFFERENCES

Definition: A disability in the child's learning process.

Author's Comment: It is important that you discuss concerns about your child's learning development and intellectual abilities with your doctor. Academic testing results and teachers' comments should also be forwarded to the doctor's office. Often, the doctor can add another dimension to educational decisions that will affect your child.

1. What are the possible causes for this condition?

Learning difference or disability is a term to describe a variety of learning problems. Children with a learning difference may have trouble with reading, writing, listening, speaking, reasoning, or doing math. The causes of learning differences are not always obvious. There may be a family history of learning issues, some children who were born prematurely have learning problems, or a childhood injury or illness may cause learning differences (for example, head injury or meningitis).

2. What can be done to remedy it?

First, talk to your child's teacher and your pediatrician if you are concerned about a learning problem in your child. Schools are mandated to help all children with learning differences at no cost to parents. Formal evaluation is required to define the problem. Your pediatrician may want to test your child's vision and hearing. At times, an evaluation by a specialist in developmental pediatrics, a psychologist, or child neurologist is needed.

Once evaluation is complete, your child may be eligible to receive special educational services to help him or her succeed in school. Modifications to your child's educational plan can help him or her master school work. These may include individual instruction, oral or untimed tests, or other accommodations to match your child's style of learning.

There is no "cure" for a learning difference. Be wary of claims that improve a child's learning through eye exercises or special glasses, diets, vitamins, or nutritional supplements. There is no evidence that these are effective.

3. How will my child be impacted educationally and career-wise in the future from this condition?

Remember that a learning difference is not an indication of your child's intellect. Most people with learning issues grow up to be very successful in life. Identifying your child's differences and obtaining the appropriate intervention as early as possible will help your child meet his or her potential. Help your child plan for the future by encouraging him or her to make choices during high school according to his or her interests and aptitude. Take advantage of school programs that teach decision making and job skills to help develop your child's abilities.

4. Will my child need to attend remedial classes or a school that specializes in these kinds of disorders?

Depending on the result of your child's learning evaluation, an Individualized Educational Plan will be developed to help promote your child's academic success. The plan may suggest resource classes, which provide more individualized instruction in core classes. Speech or occupational therapy may be recommended to help with language or writing skills. Most students can be accommodated in a regular educational setting with appropriate supports. Private schools developed for children with learning differences are available but are not necessary to meet a child's educational needs.

5. How will my child be limited in the future in regard to activity participation?

Your child's participation in physical and social activities should not be limited by having a learning difference. Some children with learning problems have emotional difficulties due to their challenges at school. Support your child's self-esteem by finding activities that interest him or her and build confidence.

6. What kind of follow-up is needed?

Ongoing surveillance of your child's educational progress is provided through school reports that chart progress toward goals set in the individual education plan. As goals are met, new ones are developed. Meetings to review the educational plan are held annually, and a full reevaluation is performed every three years.

7. Do we need to see a specialist, such as an educational psychologist for further evaluation?

School districts perform educational evaluations by a team of professionals including a psychologist and other learning specialists. At times, there may be disagreement between the assessment team and parents. An independent evaluation may be requested by parents if necessary.

8. When do you wish to see my child again for this disorder?

After the initial school evaluation is complete, a copy of the report should be sent to your pediatrician's office. A meeting to discuss the results may be requested. As long as your child is performing well in school, and annual meetings with the school are successful, periodic follow-up may not be necessary. Contact your pediatrician's office if you are concerned that your child is not making adequate progress in school, or if you have difficulty securing educational services. There are special plans to accommodate children who require assistance in school but do not meet traditional criteria for enrollment in special education services.

LISA W. GENECOV, MD
Developmental Pediatrics

LEG AND FOOT STRUCTURAL DISORDERS (e.g., Bowlegs, Knock-Knees, Pigeon-Toes, Flatfeet)

Author's Comment: Many structural abnormalities that a generation ago were treated with braces and corrective shoes are now treated with watchful observation. Nonetheless, certain structural conditions do need orthopedic evaluation and corrective procedures, so always keep the doctor informed as to your concerns in this area.

1. What causes these conditions?

Most of these conditions are normal variations of growth, and most children will outgrow these conditions, specifically bowed legs, knock-knees, and pigeon-toeing or in-toeing. There often is a family history of the condition, similar to other body traits (such as hair and eye color), and it may be genetic in nature. There are some very rare bone disorders that can cause bowed legs or knock-knees, and there are some very uncommon neurological disorders that can cause in-toeing and flatfeet. Most of the time the conditions occur for no good reason and are just part of the child's makeup.

2. Will it get worse?

The natural history for knock-knees and bowed legs is that some children start out with these conditions. They can sometimes worsen until the age of two years. From two years to eight years, improvement should be seen. If bowed legs or the knock-knees worsen after the age of two years, investigation should be done to check for an underlying reason. Sometimes corrective surgery is required, but this is uncommon, and there is no rush to have it done. Corrective surgery is done usually at five to six years of age.

In-toeing or pigeon-toeing is very common and is usually due to either the hips being rotated inward, shins being inwardly rotated, or the feet turning inward. Any one or all three of these conditions can occur in any given child. The rotation of the hips causing in-toeing changes up to the age of nine years. Twisting of the shins can spontaneously improve up to the age of six years. The inward turning of the foot can improve without treatment to the age of two years.

3. Will the condition cause my child any pain or discomfort?

Bowed legs, knock-knees, pigeon-toeing, and flatfeet rarely cause children problems in terms of pain. If your child is in pain, a search needs to be made for an underlying reason. In adults who are profoundly bowlegged, knock-kneed, or flatfooted, sometimes pain can occur, but this is often due to progressive degenerative changes in the joints. This rarely occurs in children. However, one of the reasons for following children with any of these conditions is that if the condition does not improve as they grow, then corrective interventions may need to be made to prevent long-term adult disabilities.

4. Is it correctable, or is it the type of condition that my child will outgrow without outside help?

This depends on how the child grows. Within the first three to four years of life, a lot of these conditions are normal and typically will improve. After the age of three or four years these conditions should be clearly improving. If not, then investigations should be done to check for an underlying reason. Observation is necessary within the first three to four years of life. The family history may play a major role as well.

The arch for flatfeet continues to develop to the age of twelve years. Having a flexible flatfoot up to this age can be normal. If the child has no symptoms and his or her shoes are wearing down normally, there is no need for an orthopedist consultation. The normal shoe wear pattern is that the heel should wear on the outside corner, not the inside corner.

Knock-knees and bowed legs improve up to four years of age. Whatever your child's pattern is at the age of eight years is what he or she will keep unless surgery is warranted. With in-toeing the hips can change in rotation to the age of nine years. The shins can change in rotation to the age of six years.

It is important to know a lot of professional athletes walk straight, but with running or sprinting, these athletes toe inward. Toeing inward by and of itself is not a concern unless the child has problems, such as pain or being unable to keep up with peers.

Your pediatrician is the person best trained to see initially with this problem. With his or her knowledge of you, your child, and medicine, he or she can best decide when a referral is needed. Many times your pediatrician takes great care of your child without the need for a specialist.

5. Will the condition need corrective shoes or braces to correct the problem?

If this is a condition that runs in the family, no bracing or shoe will make any difference. Studies for flatfeet have clearly proven that wearing orthotics, special shoes, or braces that support the arch do not change how the arch grows. If the child is having discomfort, these aids may help alleviate your child's symptoms. The same applies to pigeon-toeing or in-toeing. A rare form of bowed legs worsens after the age of two years and will continue to worsen without intervention; this can sometimes be improved with special leg braces. Pediatric orthopedic surgeons are trained to look for this condition by a physical examination and X rays at the age of two years.

6. Should we consult an orthopedist or a podiatrist and, if so, when?

The timing of a consultation depends largely upon the condition. For the first two to three years of life, these conditions are normal usually, and, if not causing the child any discomfort, there is no need for an orthopedist consultation, especially if you are happy with the pediatrician. The teaching and approach of these conditions is very generational. One generation ago, all of these conditions were treated with special bracing and shoe wear.

As long as the parent feels comfortable with the child's progress, there is no need for a specialist evaluation. Initially the child should be evaluated by the pediatrician to determine how serious the condition is and whether a referral to a podiatrist or orthopedic surgeon is required. Most of the time the pediatrician is well trained to manage this condition initially and will know when to refer to a specialist.

7. When do you wish to see my child again regarding this condition?

Most of the time, these conditions are assessed and reassessed during routine wellness exams at the pediatrician's office. If the condition seems to be getting worse or is causing your child to have pain or discomfort, or if you have any special concerns, you should make an appointment to see your doctor again

W. BARRY HUMENIUK, MD
Orthopedics

LYME DISEASE

Definition: A condition characterized by skin eruptions, joint aches, and sometimes heart problems caused by a certain type of tick bite.

Author's Comment: At times, this condition is difficult to diagnose and is easily confused with many other disorders that have similar symptoms. It is important to make the diagnosis as early as possible to get the appropriate treatment and to prevent complications of this disease.

1. What causes this condition, and how did my child contract it?

Lyme disease is caused by *Borrelia*, a germ that is in the spirochete classification. Borrelia is spread by tick bites. Only certain ticks carry *Borrelia*, which probably explains why almost all cases of Lyme disease occur in only a few parts of the U.S.: New England and the Mid-Atlantic East Coast, the upper Midwest, and the West Coast. Very few cases occur in the rest of the U.S. Since ticks are mainly out in the spring and summer, these are the seasons when most cases occur.

2. What symptoms might we expect to see during the natural course of this disorder?

Early in the course of Lyme disease, a very distinct type of rash usually occurs at the site of the tick bite and is often accompanied by fever, malaise, headache, and muscle aches. This is known as the early localized stage of Lyme disease.

Another stage, known as the early disseminated stage, may show itself a few weeks later as several of the skin rash lesions, along with weakness of facial muscles (due to involvement of one of the nerves that controls the facial muscles), conjunctivitis (red eyes), meningitis (manifested by headache, stiff neck), pains in the joints and muscles, and fatigue. Children who are not treated with antibiotics can go on to get arthritis, manifested by swelling and redness of one or more joints, and occasionally, by inflammation of the heart, which is much less common.

The late stage of Lyme disease includes arthritis of a few joints and some involvement of certain nerves.

3. What are the complications that can occur?

Arthritis is a common complication, and carditis (inflammation of the heart) is much less common but can occur in a small percentage of untreated children.

4. What treatment can be employed?

Antibiotics are effective in most cases. For children under eight years of age, amoxicillin is usually prescribed, and for children eight years and older, doxycycline is often used. Other antibiotics are sometimes used, depending on the symptoms and stage of the infection.

5. Are there any side effects from the treatment, and is the treatment always successful?

The usual side effects of antibiotics apply to treatment of this infection as well. The treatment is usually effective, and the earlier the stage of the disease, the more effective the treatment is. The treatment gets rid of the *Borrelia*, but sometimes the symptoms can persist for a few weeks.

6. What period of time will my child be out of school, and what kind of activity restrictions will need to be imposed?

Your child should be able to return to school as soon as he or she feels up to it. The only restrictions are those that the particular symptoms might require.

7. What can we expect as a long-term outcome from this disorder?

It depends on the stage of the infection at the time of treatment. For most cases of early stage treatment, a full recovery is common. For children with severe arthritis, the recovery usually takes longer but is often complete.

8. Do we need to consult a specialist and, if so, when and what kind?

That depends on the symptoms and the stage of the disease. Your physician can advise you about whether seeing a specialist is necessary. The laboratory testing for Lyme disease is difficult to do accurately. Many people have been told that they had Lyme disease on the basis of tests that were inaccurate. A specialist may be able to help in interpreting results of testing if your pediatrician has questions about this.

9. What symptoms would warrant getting back in touch with you immediately?

Worsening of the joint symptoms or neurologic symptoms, or changes in the mental status would warrant reevaluation. If the symptoms do not improve after treatment, evaluation for other possible causes of the symptoms may be warranted.

10. What kind of follow-up will be needed in the future?

That depends on the stage of Lyme disease in which your child was treated, and how he or she has responded. Your physician can help with guidance on follow-up.

GREGORY R. ISTRE, MD
Infectious Diseases

LYMPH NODE ENLARGEMENT
(Lymphadenopathy)

Definition: Enlarged lymph nodes (glands)

Author's Comment: Swollen glands in the neck are a common finding in many otherwise normal children. Nonetheless, if you notice the sudden appearance of swollen glands or the glands appear larger than you think they should be, it is advisable to have the condition evaluated by the doctor for some possible underlying disease.

1. What causes this condition, and how did my child develop it?

Lymph nodes are little glands that are scattered throughout the body. Lymph nodes occur in the neck, over and under the collar bones, in the arm pits, in the chest, abdomen, and in the groin area. Lymph nodes play an important part in your child's immune system and in the ability to fight infection. One of the roles of the lymph node is to act like a filter, or a little vacuum cleaner. When an infection occurs in the blood, or on the skin, the germs that are in the blood are often cleared and filtered out by the lymph nodes. When this happens, the lymph nodes may become enlarged. Sometimes, so many germs can get into a lymph node that the lymph nodes themselves can become infected. Enlarged lymph nodes is a very common finding in children. In greater than 95 percent of cases, this is caused by infection.

2. What tests need to be performed to better define this disorder?

In most cases of lymph node enlargement, no tests are necessary. Usually, the doctor will recommend close observation. Sometimes a physician will recommend antibiotics. On some occasions, the physician may order blood tests in order to better determine the exact cause of lymph node infection.

3. Can this condition lead to something more serious?

Yes. If a lymph node becomes infected and it is not treated, this can lead to a more serious infection under the skin.

4. What is the treatment for this disorder?

In general, antibiotics will be sufficient to treat any infection of the lymph node. However, it is important to realize that antibiotics are not always used for enlarged lymph nodes. If a lymph node is enlarged because a child has a viral infection, antibiotics will not be helpful. Therefore, it is up to the judgment of the physician whether or not lymph nodes require treatment. If a physician prescribes antibiotics and the lymph node does not improve, then sometimes it is necessary to do a biopsy of the lymph node, or to remove the lymph node in order to examine the lymph node under the microscope.

On some occasions, a lymph node may be enlarged due to a cause other than infection. In less than 5 percent of children with enlarged lymph nodes, there may be some underlying more serious problems such as a type of cancer. Again, it is important to realize that the great majority of children with enlarged lymph nodes do not have cancer. However, a lymph node that is continuing to enlarge over a period of a few weeks, or children with multiple enlarged lymph nodes, may have a more serious underlying condition and a biopsy of the lymph node may be required.

5. If medicines are to be used, what side effects can occur?

If a physician decides that medications are to be used for the treatment of lymph node enlargement, most likely the physician will prescribe some form of antibiotic. Antibiotics are usually well tolerated in children, though some children can be allergic to antibiotics, and some children can develop diarrhea with antibiotics. More serious reactions to antibiotics can occur, but these are not common. Your physician should review with you the potential side effects of any antibiotic.

6. How long can we expect the lymph nodes to remain enlarged?

In general, enlarged lymph nodes will resolve and get smaller within a few weeks. In certain circumstances, once a lymph node becomes infected and enlarged, it may remain slightly enlarged for many, many years. A lymph node that has been enlarged for many, many years is almost never a concern. However, a lymph node that is continuing to enlarge over a period of several weeks and not responding to antibiotic therapy is a cause for concern.

7. Are there any complications that we should look for?

Any lymph node that is enlarged and that is also tender with any redness on the surface of the skin is a complication that should be brought to the attention of the physician.

8. When do you wish to see my child again regarding this disorder?

Most children who come to the pediatrician with enlarged lymph nodes will not need to be seen again for this disorder, since most of the time the disorder will resolve by itself. If the physician feels that antibiotics are required, then often the physician will request that your child return for another examination after the antibiotics are completed.

CARL LENARSKY, MD

Hematology

MENINGITIS

Definition: Inflammation of the lining of the brain caused by infection.

Author's Comment: This disease, if caused by a bacteria, can be devastating and requires aggressive medical treatment. Fortunately, we see a lot less of it since the routine administration of certain vaccines (the hemophillus influenzae and pneumococcal vaccines). Viral meningitis is usually much less serious.

1. What causes this condition, and how did my child contract it?

Meningitis can have many causes, including infection from microorganisms such as bacteria, viruses, fungi, and parasites. The two most common causes of bacterial meningitis are *Streptococcus pneumoniae* (pneumococcus) and *Neisseria meningitidis* (meningococcus). The remainder of this section will refer specifically to bacterial meningitis from one of these bacteria. A significant percentage of healthy individuals harbor one of these bacteria in their nose or throat. A "colonized" individual may pass the bacteria to another person via respiratory secretions. Not every child who becomes colonized will become ill, though, and only a very small number will develop meningitis.

2. How serious is it?

Bacterial meningitis is a very serious, potentially life-threatening disease, with a mortality rate of approximately 5 percent to 10 percent.

3. Is it contagious and, if so, for how long and how is it spread?

Meningococcal meningitis is contagious enough to warrant special precautions, as described in question #7. A child with this disease is felt to be contagious until antibiotics have been given for about twenty-four hours.

4. What is the treatment, and is hospitalization necessary?

Children with suspected or proven bacterial meningitis are admitted to the hospital and observed carefully, often in a pediatric intensive care unit. Antibiotics are the mainstay of therapy. Other treatment is tailored to each child's unique circumstances.

5. Are there any side effects to the treatment?

Serious adverse effects from the antibiotics used to treat meningitis are uncommon.

6. Do we need to consult an infectious disease specialist?

When bacterial meningitis is especially serious or complicated, consultation with a pediatric infectious disease specialist should be considered.

7. What advice should be given to people who have had recent contact with my child?

Individuals who have been in close contact with a child with meningococcal meningitis are at significant risk of becoming ill as well. After the diagnosis is confirmed, the public health department is notified. Officials investigate the situation and determine which people may benefit from preventive antibiotics. Concerned individuals with questions should contact their public health department. When pneumococcal meningitis is diagnosed, special precautions are not necessary.

8. Will this condition cause any long-term residual effects?

Of children with bacterial meningitis, approximately 10 percent to 20 percent of survivors have significant, long-term complications, such as deafness, seizures, developmental delay, weakness or paralysis, or blindness.

9. When will my child be able to resume normal activities?

Recovery in children with bacterial meningitis varies greatly and depends on the degree of illness and the occurrence of any complications. A child is usually allowed to resume activities as able, without restriction.

10. What kind of follow-up is needed?

Outpatient follow-up is individualized. Some children may need routine checkups only. However, if complications have occurred, children may benefit from follow-up with specialists, such as audiologists, neurologists, developmental pediatricians, physical therapists, and occupational therapists. Your primary care physician usually coordinates any specialized care.

STUART W. EHRETT, MD
Infectious Diseases

MENSTRUATION–ONSET
(Menarche)

Definition: **The onset of menstruation.**

Author's Comment: Some girls have heard a lot about menarche and menstruation from their parents, friends, or other sources. Other girls know very little about menarche and menstruation. In either case, the doctor's office is a good place to ask questions, dispel myths, and divide fact from fiction with regard to menarche and other pubertal changes.

1. What is the best way to explain to my child what is happening to her body?

Menarche is one of the events involved in puberty. The changes that occur during puberty occur over a period of time, and the conversation explaining these changes should also probably take place over a period of time. Rather than one big talk, a series of conversations is probably more effective and less overwhelming. Take advantage of opportunities as they arise to talk about the changes that occur during puberty.

In discussing menarche, it is important to stress how this event is a normal part of growing up. The age and maturity of your child will dictate how much detail to include in your explanation. A basic explanation of menarche and the menstrual cycle could be something like the following:

> The changes that are occurring in your body are a normal part of growing up and changing from a child to a young woman. Women have a cycle of hormones that occurs each month. Each month, the brain produces hormones that give signals to the ovaries. The ovaries then make hormones that stimulate the lining of the uterus (womb) to become thick for a potential pregnancy. One ovary will eventually release an egg (ovulation). If the egg is fertilized (meets up with a sperm), the fertilized egg will settle in the lining of the uterus and begin to develop into a baby. If the egg is not fertilized, the egg and lining will slough off, resulting in the bleeding that is recognized as menstruation.

2. Are there any teaching aids available that may further help her understand?

Fortunately, there are now entire sections in the bookstore or library that address adolescent topics including the changes in the body associated with puberty and menarche. It may be helpful to pick up one of these books in order to better illustrate the anatomy involved in the menstrual cycle. These books also provide written information your child can read as a supplement to your conversations. One book that is particularly well written for adolescents is The "What's Happening to My Body?" Book for Girls by Lynda Madaras. It is a good idea to first read any material you plan to give to your child to make sure it agrees with your beliefs and what you want your child to know.

3. What should my daughter know specifically to aid in her hygiene?

It is important for girls and women to regularly change their pads or tampons. Toxic shock syndrome (TSS) is a potentially serious bacterial infection that is very rare but correlated with tampon use, particularly highly absorbent tampons. Therefore, girls should change their tampons every four to six hours during the day. Pads and tampons should also be changed regularly for better general hygiene and to reduce the risk of girls "bleeding through" the pad or tampon and onto their clothes. Douching should be avoided because it alters the natural pH in the vagina and can result in an overgrowth of bacteria or yeast, resulting in vaginal infections. There is also some evidence that douching can increase the susceptibility to sexually transmitted diseases.

4. How do I help her deal with the psychological aspects of this developmental stage?

If a girl is the first of her friends to start her period, it can be more challenging psychologically. On the other hand, if a girl is the only one in her group to not yet have her period, she can feel left out. At this stage of development, it is very hard to be different from one's peers. It is important to stress that menarche can occur at different ages in different girls, but that eventually every girl will start her period. Even if your child is earlier or later in this process than her friends, they will all eventually undergo menarche and the changes associated with puberty. Being open to talking about puberty and answering your daughter's questions will help her deal with the changes her body is undergoing. You can also help emphasize how these changes are a normal part of growing up, which can be very reassuring for your child.

5. Should I expect any personality changes?

The hormones involved during puberty and menarche can be associated with increased mood swings. Some girls are particularly moody for the week or two prior to their periods. It can be helpful to track mood changes. If these changes occur outside of the two weeks prior to the period, they are probably not attributable to the menstrual cycle. In addition, true personality changes or persistent depression are more than what would be expected with hormonal fluctuations of the menstrual cycle.

6. How regular should menstrual cycles be following menarche?

In the first year or two after menarche, periods can be very irregular because the hormone system that controls ovulation and menstruation is immature. However, cycles should then become regular. Even in these first years after menarche when cycles can be irregular, evaluation by a doctor is warranted if cycles are more frequent than every three weeks or less frequent than every three months.

7. When do you think it would be appropriate for her to see a gynecologist?

It is appropriate to see a gynecologist for irregular cycles or painful cramps during the menstrual cycle. Also, if a young woman is sexually active, she needs a yearly pelvic exam, screening for sexually transmitted diseases, and discussion of contraception.

KELLI WATKINS, MD
Gynecology

MOLE
(Pigmented Nevus)

Definition: A pigmented (brown) spot or bump on the skin.

Author's Comment: Moles are common among children. Nonetheless, a mole that changes in character or is painful should be brought to the attention of the doctor.

1. Is this condition in any way dangerous?

Although some moles are annoying or unsightly, most moles in children are not dangerous. Nevertheless, some moles can become abnormal and may develop into melanoma, a serious and potentially deadly type of skin cancer. Although melanoma is becoming more common in adults, it is still rare in children. Blistering sunburns and use of indoor tanning beds increase the risk of getting melanoma and should be avoided.

Since increased lifetime sun exposure and past sunburns increase the risk of melanoma, routine use of sunscreens, sun-protective clothing (long sleeves, hats), and avoidance of the more intense midday sun is highly recommended. Although melanoma is scary and we should watch for it, the majority of moles in children are just fine and do not require any treatment at all.

2. What is the possibility that it might become malignant?

Only 2 percent of all melanomas appear during childhood. The risk increases in the teenage years but is still lower relative to adults. Although the childhood risk of a mole becoming malignant is low, some children are at higher risk than others. Two of the more common risk factors are genetics and the presence of giant congenital moles (large moles that are present since birth). If there are people in the immediate family with either numerous larger, odd-looking moles (dysplastic moles) or a past melanoma, then their siblings and children have a higher chance of developing dysplastic moles or melanoma during their lifetime.

Large ("giant" or "bathing trunk") moles that have been present since birth are more likely to develop melanoma than moles that appear later in childhood. Most of the childhood melanomas occur within giant congenital moles. These children should have their moles looked at least one to two times a year, more often in the first few years of life or if changes are noted, or parents may wish to consider surgical removal of the mole.

Increased sun exposure and multiple blistering sunburns during childhood also increase the likelihood of developing a malignant mole. This is particularly true for children with fair skin and an inability to tan. Lastly, children with genetic skin conditions causing extreme sun sensitivity and children who have suppressed immune systems (due to either genetic conditions or chemotherapy or transplant medications) may be at increased risk.

3. What changes would I look for that might indicate something worrisome is occurring?

Children get new moles all the time, and their moles change in size and color with age, so it can be difficult to know which changes are fine and which changes are not. Some changes are expected. In preadolescents, for example, it is common for moles to become darker, more raised, and for dark hairs to appear in the center. Just because a mole is hairy or becomes raised does not mean that the mole is bad.

Worrisome signs include changes in color or shape that occur in an asymmetric or off-center fashion. A rule of thumb is that if you draw a line down the center of a mole, the two halves should look the same, and one half should be a mirror image of the other. If one half of the mole has a bump or color change that is not on the other half, then that mole needs to be checked. Other causes for concern are moles that are painful, itchy, or that bleed for no reason.

4. When should we consider having a mole removed?

If your doctor sees a mole that is odd or not symmetric in color or shape, then he or she may recommend removal to determine if it is abnormal. Another reason for removal may be if the mole is symptomatic (tender, bleeding, or itchy). Removal should also be considered for larger moles that were present at birth since they are at increased risk for malignancy, but removal is not mandatory unless abnormal features are present.

Removing all of a person's moles does not eliminate his or her lifetime risk of melanoma, since melanomas frequently appear at sites where there was no mole, so total body mole removal is not recommended for anyone. You should also be aware that it is impossible to completely remove a mole without leaving a scar, and scars do not always heal well. This should be kept in mind if your child wants a mole removed just because he or she does not like it—he or she may be more unhappy with a scar. Any mole that is removed—no matter the reason—should be sent to the lab (preferably to a skin pathologist or dermatopathologist) for evaluation.

5. Do we need to see a dermatologist?

If you or your pediatrician are concerned by the changes in a mole, then it may need to be evaluated by a dermatologist. Dermatology consultation is also recommended if your family has a history of moles that grow abnormally (dysplastic moles) or melanoma or if your child was born with a large mole. Dermatologists have a lot of training and experience in the evaluation of moles, which helps in the early detection of abnormal changes. They are also very comfortable performing skin biopsies, if this is needed, and know how to interpret the pathology findings after a mole is removed. Because melanoma risk starts to rise in the teenage years and because teens may not allow parents to look at their skin, it is a good idea for all teenagers or young adults to have at least one total body mole evaluation by a dermatologist.

6. What kind of follow-up is needed for this condition?

Most moles require no follow-up, unless concerning changes are noted. If your child has a giant congenital mole or another risk factor for malignancy, then yearly mole evaluations would be recommended. During the first few years of life, giant congenital moles may need to be evaluated every three to six months. More frequent evaluations may also be needed if your child had a melanoma or if he or she has a genetic condition causing severe sun sensitivity.

K. ROBIN CARDER, MD
Dermatology

MONONUCLEOSIS

Definition: An acute viral illness that usually gets better on its own, characterized by fever, fatigue, swollen tonsils, enlarged lymph nodes, and sometimes enlargement of the spleen.

Author's Comment: This condition, referred to as the "kissing disease," can be contracted through transfer of human saliva. It is very common in teens and needs close follow-up with the doctor. Generally, it takes quite awhile for the child's energy to fully return.

1. What causes this condition, and how did my child contract it?

Mononucleosis, also called infectious mononucleosis or mono, is most commonly caused by a virus called Epstein-Barr virus (EBV). Occasionally, similar symptoms can be caused by other viruses, such as cytomegalovirus (CMV) and other germs, but the majority are due to EBV.

Symptoms can vary from mild or no symptoms to more severe symptoms, but most commonly they include fever, enlarged lymph nodes, sore throat and tonsillitis, rash, and enlarged spleen. For some reason, children with mononucleosis are prone to get a rash if they take ampicillin or amoxicillin, even if they are not allergic to those antibiotics, so it is best to avoid those antibiotics if a person has mononucleosis.

Other more severe symptoms may occur in a small proportion of children who contract EBV. The typical age to contract mononucleosis is adolescence, but it can occur at any age. Symptoms seem to be worst in adolescent and adult persons, and less severe in younger children. A person contracts EBV infection from another person who has the infection. It is usually spread by contact with saliva and occasionally from blood transfusions.

2. Is it contagious, and, if so, what can I do to prevent its spread?

It is mildly contagious, but only from direct contact with saliva or respiratory secretions, or rarely from blood transfusions.

3. What complications of this condition should I watch for?

The most frequent complications arise from the enlargement of the spleen or the tonsils. Because the spleen is enlarged, it can rupture more easily, so contact sports should be avoided until the spleen is back to normal size. The enlargement of the tonsils can result in noisy breathing or, if severe enough, in difficulty with breathing.

4. Are there any medicines used to treat the disease?

There is no medication that has been shown to be effective in treating mononucleosis.

5. Should the use of steroids be considered to shrink the size of the tonsils and make my child feel better?

Steroids are usually reserved for use in severe cases of enlargement of the tonsils to the point that the child has trouble breathing, For most cases of mononucleosis, steroids are not used.

6. How long is the condition contagious, and how do I keep it from spreading?

Mononucleosis is only mildly contagious at its peak, but a person with mononucleosis continues to have the virus in his or her secretions for a few weeks after the initial symptoms. Since it is mainly spread through secretions such as saliva, avoiding contact with saliva and respiratory secretions and good handwashing are adequate to prevent spread.

7. How long does the illness last?

The symptoms may last for several days, or up to a few weeks. The typical adolescent or adult who gets mononucleosis feels sick for several weeks and is tired for a month or more.

8. How long does my child need to stay completely away from all physical exercise, and what is the timetable for resuming activities and returning to school?

Stay away from contact sports until the spleen enlargement has completely resolved. Other types of physical exercise can be done as tolerated, but fatigue is a common symptom that can be present for several weeks. Your child can return to school as soon as he or she can tolerate it.

9. What advice should be given to people who have been recently in contact with my child?

Because this is a very common infection and many people have had the infection in the past, and because it is not easily transmitted to others, the chance of another person getting mononucleosis from your child is low. Nevertheless, persons who had contact with saliva from an infected person could get mononucleosis, so they should let their physician know if they develop symptoms of mononucleosis. But keep in mind that there is no treatment for the infection, and it runs its course after several days or weeks.

10. Can this condition recur or become chronic?

Only in rare cases does mononucleosis recur or become chronic.

11. When do you wish to see my child again for follow-up?

If the spleen was enlarged, then it should be checked again, and contact sports avoided until your physician gives the okay to resume. If your child develops difficulty breathing or becomes sicker, or if the symptoms do not get better after a few weeks, you should see your physician again.

GREGORY R. ISTRE, MD
Infectious Diseases

MOOD DISORDER
(e.g., Depression, Anxiety, Mania)

Author's Comment: These types of disorders seem to occur with increasing frequency in pediatric practices. If you suspect your child has a mood disorder, discuss it with the doctor. These conditions, if severe and left untreated, can be quite disruptive to a child's happiness and family life.

1. Why do children experience this type of disorder?

Mood and anxiety disorders are thought to be serious medical conditions that do have a genetic predisposition. In other words, a strong family history is an indicator that a child may have a vulnerability to develop depression, anxiety, or mania under duress. Anxiety and depressive disorders are quite prevalent in our society but must be differentiated from adjustment disorders or disorders based on reactions to life situations.

2. How serious do you think this disorder is in my child?

By definition, a mood or an anxiety disorder can become serious if it becomes disruptive to that child's capacity to function effectively. Our goal as parents is not only to see that our children have a happy and productive childhood but also to see that they develop the appropriate coping skills to deal with social and academic stressors. If those coping skills appear to be severely impaired, then one must consider the "episode" to be a serious one.

3. Is the disorder genetic, or is it environmentally acquired?

Most mood disorders are thought to have a strong genetic basis. However, environmental factors clearly play a role. Living in a family environment in which a child is neglected or emotionally, physically, or sexually abused would represent obvious causes and risk factors for development of a mood or anxiety disorder.

4. How can I tell whether this is a phase or a long-term condition?

Typically, we consider adjustment disorders to be of six months duration or less. An adjustment disorder would display symptoms of anxiety or depression that follow a significant stressor such as a move, divorce, loss of a family member, or other traumatic event. However, beyond six months the concern would quickly develop that a more specific mood episode could be developing that warrants further attention.

5. What can I do as a parent to make it better?

The most important intervention that a parent can make is to have an awareness of any early symptom developments. Be on the lookout for issues such as changes in sleep and appetite patterns, dropping grades, increased isolation and withdrawal from the child's usual activities, or changes in his or her behavioral pattern.

6. Does the condition warrant consulting a psychiatrist or psychologist?

Consultation with a psychologist or psychiatrist is warranted if the child appears to be struggling in his or her ability to implement good coping strategies beyond the typical "adjustment phase" when a stressor has occurred within the family system. Academic decline or withdrawal or isolation from parents, which makes it difficult for parents to gauge the severity of a mood or anxiety episode, would warrant an initial evaluation with a psychologist. Psychiatric care might be appropriate if there is a strong suspicion that a family history of depressive or anxiety disorder is beginning to show itself, with an impact on sleep, appetite, and energy level changes.

7. Is there any medicine that can be used to improve this condition, and, if so, are there any side effects?

There is a long list of medications that can improve depressive anxiety and other mood disorders. Many of these medications, however, have been closely scrutinized out of concerns about safety and side effects. In particular, the FDA has been closely monitoring the use of antidepressant medications in younger populations because of the side effects. If medication is being considered, consultation with a child psychiatrist would be most appropriate. Certain antidepressant medications can be very beneficial and even "life saving" but need to be monitored by a professional who is very comfortable in discussing therapeutic benefits and side effects.

8. When do you wish to see my child again for this condition?

Often children need to be seen quite frequently as they are working through a depressive or anxiety or manic episode to ensure that there is no further decline in the level of functioning. Usually, weekly therapy is appropriate and, if psychiatric or medication intervention has been started, visits are very frequent in the initial phase of treatment to ascertain that there are no side effects and that good therapeutic benefits are taking place.

DANTE BURGOS, MD
Psychiatry

MOUTH INFECTION
(Stomatitis)

Definition: **Inflammation of the mouth.**

Author's Comment: This condition can be very unpleasant and painful for a child. A parent has to be quite resourceful in employing a treatment program that affords the child some comfort and relief.

1. What is the cause of this condition, and how did my child contract it?

Mouth ulcers or inflammation of the mouth lining (stomatitis) are often caused by viral infections, particularly *herpes simplex* virus and enteroviruses. Apthous stomatitis is a condition where isolated shallow mouth ulcers appear but do not have any infectious cause. Stomatitis from viral infections usually occurs in children less than four years of age. In addition to painful mouth ulcers, children with these viral infections also may have high fever and fussiness. These viruses are usually spread by direct contact with an infected person's saliva.

2. Is it contagious and, if so, for how long?

Children are contagious for the first five to seven days of the illness, shedding the virus in saliva. The mouth lesions and pain can take two weeks to completely resolve. Children with viral stomatitis who do not have control over their oral secretions should not attend daycare, and toys and utensils that come into contact with their saliva should be thoroughly washed. They can be allowed to return to daycare five to seven days after the first mouth lesions appear, if no new lesions are developing.

3. How is it spread?

These viral infections are spread by direct contact. Herpes simplex viruses can be spread from the mouth to other parts of the body, and children who are prone to putting their fingers in their mouths can spread vesicles to their fingers. Enteroviral infections are commonly spread by the fecal-oral route, so handwashing is essential to prevent spread to others in the household, particularly with diaper changes.

4. What is the treatment, and how effective is it?

Stomatitis is usually not treated in patients without immune problems, since the illness resolves by itself over a week or so. In severe cases of herpes stomatitis, your physician may recommend a prescription oral antiviral medication called acyclovir, which may be of some benefit in decreasing the severity and duration of symptoms.

5. Are there any side effects that can occur from the treatment?

Oral acyclovir is generally well tolerated but can cause some nausea.

6. What can be done to relieve the symptoms?

Ibuprofen or acetaminophen may help with pain and fever. Your physician may also recommend anesthetic mouth rinses, which can provide additional short-term pain control. Encourage your child to drink lots of cold fluids and eat popsicles, which can also soothe the pain.

7. Can this condition recur, and, if so, are there any ways to prevent it?

Although mouth ulcers caused by enteroviruses do not recur, stomatitis from herpes infection can recur. Even after resolution of the mouth ulcers, the herpes virus will remain within the nerves of the mouth for life. Recurrences of herpetic lesions in the mouth and on the lips (cold sores), commonly occur during times of stress, illness, or mouth injury. The recurrent flare-ups are typically milder and become less frequent with age. If herpetic recurrences are very frequent, your physician may recommend trying antiviral medication to prevent or suppress further episodes.

8. When do I call you back if the condition does not seem to be getting better?

The most serious complication of stomatitis is dehydration caused by mouth pain and a child's reluctance to drink. Occasionally children may need to be admitted to the hospital for rehydration with intravenous fluids. You should contact your doctor if your child is not drinking enough.

9. When do you wish to see my child again regarding this illness?

Unless there are complications, your child usually does not need to be seen again for this illness.

WENDY CHUNG, MD
Infectious Diseases

NECK MUSCLE CONTRACTION
(Torticollis)

Definition: **A contracted state of the neck muscle producing tilting of the head.**

Author's Comment: This condition is frequently seen in early infancy. Parents should follow the exercises that the doctor prescribes to treat this condition, even though the exercises are unpleasant for the infant. If treated, you seldom see an older child with a significant residual problem from this condition.

1. What is the cause of this condition, and how did my child develop it?

No one is exactly sure what causes muscular torticollis, but there are a number of theories. The most common theory is that when the infant is still in the womb his or her head is tilted to one side for a considerable period of time, leading to the development of shorter neck muscles on that side. Another theory is that some injury occurs while in the womb, or during delivery, that leads to muscle injury, and subsequent scarring, preventing the muscle from lengthening naturally. Finally, there may be a fusion of the neck vertebrae that prevents the neck from straightening.

2. What kind of treatment is recommended, and how effective is it?

For milder cases of muscular torticollis, no treatment is necessary. Infants are extremely curious about the world around them and will stretch their neck muscles out by themselves. For moderate cases, where there is more limitation in neck movement, physical therapy is recommended to additionally stretch the neck muscles. Parents are cautioned not to let this therapy cause any significant discomfort, because it might interfere with parental bonding. For severe limitations of neck movement, botulinum toxin may be injected into the muscle to prevent spasm and help to lengthen the muscle. After a year of age, if significant head tilting persists, surgery may be recommended to release the tightened muscle.

3. Can we expect a total correction of the condition and, if so, over what period of time?

For milder cases, a total correction can be expected. As the condition worsens, it is less likely that a complete correction can be obtained. Except for the most severe cases (which often are accompanied by bony fusions of the neck vertebrae), most parents should expect to see a correction sufficient to improve the head tilt, to the point that it is not noticeable to the average person.

4. Do we need to see a surgeon or a physical therapist for this condition?

Your pediatrician is the best person to start with to determine if any treatment is necessary. Sometimes, repositioning during feeding and sleeping will be all that is necessary. As the severity increases, physical therapy, a visit to a neurologist (for botulinum toxin injections), a consultation with a pediatric orthopedic surgeon, or pediatric plastic surgeon may be necessary. In general, surgery is reserved only for the most severe cases and for children over one year of age who have not improved with more conservative therapies.

5. What kind of follow-up is needed?

As long as progress is made and your child's range of motion is improving, specific follow-up is not necessary other than routine checkups. However, if it seems that progress is halted and there are no gains in range of motion, then a follow-up is recommended and referral to a specialist is likely.

JEFFREY A. FEARON, MD
Craniofacial Surgery

NEPHRITIS

Definition: Inflammation of the kidney frequently characterized by blood in the urine.

Author's Comment: This condition can possibly lead to progressively more impaired kidney function. It needs close and sustained follow-up with the child's physician.

1. What causes this disorder, and how did my child contract it?

Nephritis means inflammation of the kidney. Inflammation of the kidney can occur following a streptococcal infection (usually a sore throat) and is termed poststreptococcal glomerulonephritis. This usually occurs two to four weeks after the streptococcal infection. Poststreptococcal glomerulonephritis is a delayed inflammatory response to leftover streptococcal germ particles. While blood pressures may be elevated in the early phase of this condition, the long-term outlook is excellent.

Other causes of nephritis are much less common and include certain systemic, chronic viral or bacterial infections, or rheumatic disorders such as lupus.

2. What are the potential complications or dangers associated with this condition?

The most immediate danger posed by nephritis is elevated blood pressure. Often a child with poststreptococcal glomerulonephritis is admitted to the hospital to control the blood pressure. Once the blood pressure is well controlled, the ultimate prognosis of this condition is excellent.

The other forms of nephritis can be complicated, not only hypertension, but also decreased kidney function and loss of protein in the urine. Modest reductions in kidney function are potentially treatable and reversible while more severe reductions of kidney function will require hospitalization and further evaluation. In some cases, a diagnostic kidney biopsy will be performed.

Nephritis is accompanied by blood and protein in the urine. Blood in the urine is not harmful per se. Loss of modest amounts of protein in the urine is usually without major symptoms. However, loss of significant urine protein can cause swelling in the body. If such swelling occurs, it is important to call your physician.

3. What tests are needed to further determine the cause of this disorder?

Your doctor will order blood and urine tests to help identify the cause of nephritis and the severity of the kidney disease. At times, a kidney ultrasound will be used to examine the size and shape of the kidneys. A kidney biopsy may be required to determine the exact cause of the nephritis. This is a procedure where a small piece of kidney tissue is obtained via a brief procedure performed under anesthesia. The kidney tissue is sent to a pathologist who will perform special tests to help determine the nature and cause of the nephritis.

4. Is there any specific treatment, and, if so, are there any potential side effects associated with the treatment?

Any specific treatments depend upon the exact cause of the nephritis and the associated symptoms. In poststreptococcal glomerulonephritis and other forms of nephritis, medical treatment is often focused upon control of blood pressure. Diuretics or other blood pressure–lowering agents may be used. In some situations where kidney function may be compromised, steroids or other similar immunosuppressive medications may be used to help suppress the kidney inflammation. These medications can potentially suppress the immune system and lead to infections. Careful monitoring of the immune system is recommended.

5. Is exercise harmful with this condition?

Exercise is not harmful in patients with nephritis. However, if your child is hypertensive, blood pressure should be well controlled before engaging in physical activity. A good general rule is to allow your child to participate in physical exercise at the level he or she feels comfortable with. It is important not to push your child past his or her level of comfort, especially when he or she recently had a period of convalescence.

6. Will there be any long-term kidney damage?

In children with poststreptococcal glomerulonephritis, there is virtually no long-term kidney damage. Full recovery is expected. However, in the other forms of nephritis, there may be varying degrees of residual kidney damage. In many children, the degree of kidney damage can be controlled with medical treatment so that further kidney injury is limited. Your pediatrician will likely refer your child to a pediatric nephrologist to monitor and treat any kidney damage. Rarely, the kidney damage can be so great that the child will need some form of dialysis to replace the kidney function.

7. Do we need to see a nephrologist (kidney specialist) and, if so, when?

Your child will be referred to a pediatric nephrologist if there is

- any question about the diagnosis;
- hypertension;
- swelling or edema;
- hematuria involves visibly bloody urine;
- reduction in kidney function.

8. Are there any restrictions—physical, dietary, or otherwise—to be imposed upon my child that might aid in the recovery process?

With regard to physical restrictions, see question #5. Dietary restrictions often involve a reduction in salt intake. A dietician will instruct your family on a low salt diet. A reduction in salt will help to control blood pressure and reduce any edema (organ swelling). With any reduction in kidney function, it is also important to adhere to a diet low in phosphate. Phosphate, which is normally excreted by the kidneys, can accumulate to harmful levels in the face of kidney disease. Foods high in phosphate include many diary products. Your child's nephrologist may prescribe medicine to be taken with meals to help reduce the absorption of dietary phosphate.

9. What signs should I look for that I need to call you back?

In children with nephritis, uncontrolled hypertension requires urgent attention. Symptoms of hypertension can include headaches and blurry vision. However, many children with moderate or even severe hypertension have few, if any, symptoms. In some situations, your physician may instruct you to measure your child's blood pressure at home. Be clear about the range of the acceptable blood pressures and call your physician if the blood pressures are either above or below the acceptable range.

You should also alert your physician should your child develop progressively more edema. Edema may be a sign of reduced kidney function or loss of protein in the urine. Your physician can evaluate the potential cause of the edema and recommend further therapy.

10. When do you wish to see my child again regarding this condition?

Children with nephritis should be periodically followed by a pediatric nephrologist. The nephrologist will assess your child's blood pressure, level of kidney function, and urinary protein losses, if any. If your child has poststreptococcal glomerulonephritis, follow-up will be required periodically for up to one year after diagnosis. During that year, your child's kidney function and urine tests will likely return to normal. With regard to the other forms of nephritis, follow-up with the nephrologist will depend upon the severity of kidney involvement.

ALBERT QUAN, MD
Nephrology

NEPHROTIC SYNDROME

Definition: Impairment of the kidney, characterized by loss of protein in the urine and generalized body swelling.

Author's Comment: This kidney disorder can be very disfiguring during episodes of flare-up coupled with the side effects of steroid treatment. It is always important for the parent to keep in mind that, if the common form of the disease is present in his or her child, these changes are usually totally reversible, and the long-term outcome is very good.

1. What causes this disorder, and how did my child contract it?

Nephrotic syndrome refers to severe loss of protein in the urine, resulting in a low blood protein level. The most common disease-causing nephrotic syndrome in children is minimal change disease. Minimal change disease usually occurs between the ages of eighteen months to eight years of age and is often preceded by a viral respiratory infection. The subsequent urinary protein loss and low blood protein leads to fluid retention in the body, which appears as swelling in the face, abdomen, and legs. The cause of minimal change disease is unknown but is easily treatable and ultimately carries a good prognosis.

In children who are under one year of age or who are in their teen years, nephrotic syndrome can be caused by very different diseases from minimal change disease. Such diseases often carry worse prognosis than minimal change disease.

2. What are the potential complications or dangers associated with this condition?

Nephrotic syndrome is complicated by overall body edema (swelling). This edema is usually seen as puffy eyes, enlarged abdomen, and swelling around the ankles. Although the edema is cosmetically disturbing, it does not pose any harm to your child. With resolution of the nephrotic syndrome, the edema will resolve.

Loss of protein from nephrotic syndrome can also suppress your child's immune system, making him or her susceptible to certain bacterial infections. It is important for your child to see a physician if you feel he or she is ill or has a fever. Earlier detection and treatment lead to better outcomes.

The natural course of minimal change disease usually includes a number of relapses. Over time, patients will have fewer relapses with eventual complete resolution. Minimal change diseases and its relapses are easily treatable with oral steroids. Other causes of nephrotic syndrome other than minimal change disease often do not respond to medical treatment and can lead to worsening of kidney function.

3. What tests are needed to further determine the cause of this disorder?

Your physician will initially order a urine test to evaluate the amount of urinary protein. In addition, your doctor may wish to obtain a twenty-four-hour urine collection to better quantify the amount of protein loss. Blood tests will be used to help identify the cause of your child's nephrotic syndrome. On occasion, your physician may refer your child to a pediatric nephrologist (kidney specialist) for a kidney biopsy to better identify the disease process involved.

4. Is there any specific treatment, and, if so, are there any potential side effects associated with the treatment?

Minimal change disease is usually treated with oral steroids over a twelve-week period. The side effects of steroids include increased appetite and weight gain, elevated blood pressure, diabetes, and mood swings. All of these side effects will remit when the steroids are discontinued. Weight gain, however, may be difficult to reverse if your child excessively consumes high calorie foods. The elevation of blood pressure and diabetes are treated with use of medications or dietary changes.

If your child has a different cause of nephrotic syndrome, your nephrologist may elect to use medications that suppress the immune system. By suppressing the immune system, it is hoped that the nephrotic syndrome will go into remission or at least be well controlled. With all medicines that suppress the immune system, your child should be brought to a physician if he or she is ill or has a fever.

5. Is exercise harmful with this condition?

Your child with may exercise as he or she pleases. However, the edema may physically limit the extent of the activity. For example, swelling in the ankles may limit the ability to run and play. In addition, steroid medication can reduce your child's stamina and endurance for strenuous physical activity.

6. Will there be any long-term kidney damage?

Minimal change disease virtually never causes any permanent kidney damage. However, other diseases associated with nephrotic syndrome can cause kidney damage. In some cases, the kidney damage may be irreversible and result in a reduced kidney function. If your child has reduced kidney function, he or she should be followed by a pediatric nephrologist to help monitor the kidney function and for any potential complications.

Some medications used to treat nephrotic syndrome can also cause kidney damage, if used for a prolonged period of time. Your nephrologist will try to limit your child's exposure to these medications and will monitor kidney function.

7. Do we need to see a nephrologist (kidney specialist), and, if so, when?

As mentioned, most children with nephrotic syndrome who are between the ages of eighteen months to eight years have minimal change disease. Many children with minimal change disease are initially diagnosed and treated by a pediatric nephrologist. Subsequent follow-up can take place with your child's nephrologist or pediatrician in uncomplicated cases. Frequent relapses of nephrotic syndrome or failure to respond to medical therapy will require consultation with a nephrologist. Also, a child with nephrotic syndrome and hypertension, or reduced kidney function, will require a visit to a nephrologist.

8. Are there any restrictions—physical, dietary, or otherwise—to be imposed upon my child that might aid in the recovery process?

There are no absolute physical restrictions per se in children with nephrotic syndrome. However, children with edema may have some modest physical limitations that will resolve after the edema goes away. Children with nephrotic syndrome should be on a low salt diet. A diet with unrestricted salt intake will exacerbate the development of edema. Dietary salt restriction may be lifted when your child's nephrotic syndrome has resolved and the steroid therapy has finished.

9. What signs should I look for that would warrant my calling you back?

You should call your physician if your child develops edema. Your child's physician will provide you with instructions regarding steroid therapy and subsequent follow-up. Do not begin steroid therapy without first consulting your physician. Should your child develop a fever, it is important to seek medical attention urgently. Children with nephrotic syndrome are immune suppressed and can develop serious bacterial infections. Your child may be hospitalized to receive antibiotics if necessary.

10. When do you wish to see my child again regarding this condition?

Children with nephrotic syndrome require periodic follow-up during their initial episode to assure an appropriate response to steroid therapy. Follow-up is also recommended during subsequent relapses. As mentioned, any child with nephrotic syndrome who has a fever requires urgent medical attention.

ALBERT QUAN, MD
Nephrology

NOSEBLEEDS

Author's Comment: This is a condition that can occur in clusters and usually resolves on its own. If your child gets frequent nosebleeds, check with your child's doctor because there could be an underlying problem.

1. What causes this condition, and how did my child develop it?

Nosebleeds are a very common condition in young children. Most children will have at least one nosebleed during their preschool years. Nosebleeds in children typically come from the front part of the nose from an area just inside the nostril on the middle portion of the nose known as the septum.

The causes of nosebleeds include the following:

- **Trauma:** The most common type of trauma is from picking the nose, putting some object in the nose, or blowing the nose too hard. Trauma can also include hits to the nose that may result in a fracture. Or, in more severe cases, a fracture of the skull can lead to a nosebleed.

- **Colds or allergies:** In a child with allergies or an infection, the lining of the nose is swollen and irritated. This can cause itching that may lead to nose picking and nosebleeds. In addition, both conditions frequently require nose blowing. If the child blows his or her nose too vigorously or sneezes too forcefully, this can lead to a nosebleed.

- **Dry air:** During the fall and winter months, the humidity level is typically very low in cold climates. The low humidity can cause the child's nose to dry out. The blood vessels on the septum are just underneath the surface and cracks from the dryness may lead to bleeding.

- **Abnormal blood clotting:** Clotting disorders can be genetic (run in families) or can be due to medications the child might be taking. A common medication taken by children that leads to abnormal blood clotting is ibuprofen. Aspirin also leads to a child's blood not clotting correctly.

- **Tumors:** Tumors are a very, very rare cause of nosebleeds in young children. Most tumors or abnormal growths in the nose that would lead to bleeding in young children are typically benign. All abnormal growths in a child's nose should be evaluated by a physician promptly. Adolescent boys can rarely develop a vascular tumor in the back of the nose that often first shows up as nosebleeds.

2. Can nosebleeds be dangerous?

Most children will have a least one nosebleed. Many children will have frequent nosebleeds, and this is not an uncommon condition. Some children will have several nosebleeds each week during their preschool and grade school years.

Nosebleeds in young children are rarely dangerous; however, they can be frightening. In addition to bright red blood coming briskly from the nose, if your child swallows blood during the nosebleed, this can lead to nausea and vomiting of blood.

The condition can be dangerous if your child has a clotting disorder or a tumor (an abnormal growth) in his or her nose.

Your child should be evaluated by a physician if he or she is having recurrent nosebleeds, you have difficulty controlling the nosebleeds, or your child has a nosebleed that you cannot control.

3. Can my child become anemic from the loss of blood?

If your child is otherwise healthy and does not have a bleeding disorder or an abnormal growth in his or her nose, it is rare that he or she would become anemic from nosebleeds.

However, if nosebleeds are not easily controlled and happen frequently, anemia can occur. It is extremely rare that your child would need a blood transfusion to replace lost blood.

4. What can I do to treat the nosebleeds when they occur?

Steps for controlling a bleeding nose:

1. **Remain calm.** If children are agitated, they may bleed more profusely than if they are calm and reassured.
2. **Elevate.** Keep the head elevated higher than the level of the heart. It is best if your child is in a sitting position with the head tilted slightly forward. Do not lay your child down flat.
3. **Clear.** Attempt to clear nose of all blood clots. If your child is old enough, have him or her blow the nose to clear the clots.
4. **Pinch.** Pinch the lower half of your child's nose (the soft part) between your thumb and the side of your index finger. Hold it firmly, almost to the point of discomfort.

5. **Press.** Press firmly with your thumb and the side of your index finger toward the face, compressing the pinched soft parts of the nose against the bones of the face.

6. **Hold.** Hold this position for a full five minutes by the clock. When you release the nose after the full five minutes, if the bleeding has not stopped, repeat steps one through five. The second time, hold the position for a full ten minutes by the clock. If, after ten more minutes of pressure, the bleeding has not stopped, call your physician or go to the nearest emergency room.

5. What can be done to prevent the nosebleeds from recurring?

Encourage your child to not pick his or her nose. Keeping the finger nails trimmed very short can help.

The best way to prevent nosebleeds is to provide humidity and moisture to the lining of the nose. This can be done by placing a pea-sized amount of lubricating ointment (such as petroleum ointment) on the end of your fingertip and then rubbing it inside the nose. In a small child, the pea-sized amount of ointment will block the nostril. The ointment can then be easily distributed by gently squeezing the soft part of the nose. This can be done as frequently as needed, usually every night at bedtime is enough.

Saline nasal spray or the use of a room humidifier during dry winter months may also help to moisten the lining of a dry nose.

If the nosebleeds persist despite these steps, you should see your child's physician. Your physician may refer your child to a specialist for invasive measures to prevent the recurrence of nosebleeds.

6. Do we need to see an ear, nose, and throat specialist and, if so, when?

If your child's nosebleeds do not improve with the earlier steps or cannot be controlled with a nose pinch and pressure, then your physician may refer you to see a specialist.

The specialist may examine your child's nose with an endoscope (a tube with a light for seeing inside the nose) to identify the source of the bleeding.

The specialist may control the nosebleed with packing or cauterization of the blood vessel. If your child is old enough to have the nosebleeds controlled while awake, the physician will cauterize the vessel(s) in clinic. Cauterization done while a child is awake is done after the application of a topical local anesthetic agent. To cauterize the blood vessel, a chemical substance (silver nitrate) is used to burn and seal the vessels and stop the bleeding. Young children often will not tolerate cauterization under local anesthesia in the clinic. In these cases the specialist may recommend that your child undergo a general anesthetic to control the bleeding.

7. When do you wish to see my child again regarding this condition?

Your child may not need to be seen again if the nosebleeds stop occurring after the use of ointments or other humidification.

Your child should be seen by his or her physician again if he or she continues to have nosebleeds after an appropriate trial of humidification therapy, if the blood is coming only from your child's mouth, or if he or she is coughing or vomiting blood or brown material that looks like coffee grounds.

PAUL W. BAUER, MD
Otolaryngology

OBESITY

Definition: A complex chronic condition of being
grossly overweight due to the excessive
accumulation of fat in the body.

Author's Comment: This is a challenging problem. Children today are three times more likely to be obese than they were forty years ago. The problem is multifaceted, and the treatment must come with the family working closely with the physician and possibly other specialists.

1. What are the likely factors that contribute to my child's weight problem?

Obesity exists when food, or calories consumed, exceeds the activity level, or calories used, of the child. Added to this are family weight trends, school, and social environments. Most children with obesity simply eat too many calories for their energy needs. Many children have regular access to poor food choices such as fast, high-fat, high-sugar, low-quality foods. As little as a 5 percent increase in daily calorie increase can result in significant weight gain when measured over the span of months to years. Finally, inactivity from watching television, playing video games and computer games, or limited opportunity for regular play and exercise will decrease the calories used by the child.

2. Are there any tests that need to be done to explore the possibility of an underlying cause?

In most cases, the history and physical exam of the child will give your doctor the information he or she needs to diagnose childhood obesity. A comparison of your child's weight to height for age (the body mass index or BMI) can define the degree of obesity. In rare circumstances, an endocrine (hormonal) or metabolic evaluation may be in order. With the combination of some simple blood and urine tests, these conditions can be eliminated from consideration.

3. What are the potential problems and complications that this condition can cause for my child?

Obesity can involve almost every organ system in the body. The most common complications include Type 2 (insulin-resistant) diabetes, heart disease, fatty liver, elevated cholesterol, orthopedic abnormalities, obstructive sleep apnea, and female reproductive problems. Most of these are reversible by addressing the obesity early.

4. What can be done to help correct or counteract this condition?

Education about age-appropriate diets and calorie requirements is the first step to correcting the problem. Monitoring fast food intake, as well as limiting prolonged periods of inactivity all need to be addressed as family lifestyle changes. Many obese children will also have overweight or obese parents. In most instances, the child will only have success in weight management if the whole family is invested to reduce weight together. The Centers for Disease Control (CDC), as well as multiple other government and private organizations have websites designed to help get you started.

5. Is there anything that we, as parents, should do?

Recognize that obesity is not primarily a social or emotional statement about your child; rather, realize that this condition can have a real, long-lasting, permanent effects on your child's physical and mental well-being. Taking an active role in addressing the problem is extremely important for success. Statistically, obese children are more likely to be obese adults. They are also much more likely to have obese children of their own. Obesity can not only reduce the quality and duration of life but also the anticipated increase in health care costs and decreased ability to work could leave your child with a lifetime of financial and social disadvantage.

6. Do you think we should consult a specialty clinic, psychologist, or dietician?

If initial attempts at controlling excessive weight gain are unsuccessful, then specialty help may be needed. A psychologist can help with self-image and motivation issues, as well as complex family dynamics. A dietician can help a family choose age-appropriate choices for the children and give guidelines for situations with school lunches and eating out. In some situations, obesity-related specialty clinics may be useful for comprehensive care, but widespread availability for children is limited.

7. What kind of follow-up will be needed in the future?

Usually, routine visits with your pediatrician or family doctor will suffice once your child's weight has stabilized. Ideal body weight can easily be followed by tracking the height and weight.

KENDALL O. BROWN, MD
Gastroenterology

PIN WORMS
(Enterobiasis)

Definition: A relatively common childhood infection caused by a smallish roundworm that is passed from child to child and that inhabits the intestines of humans.

Author's Comment: This is the most common parasitic worm infection in humans. Most parents are aghast when first sighting these disgusting little worms. Fortunately, in the vast majority of cases, the sight of the worms is much worse than the condition itself as these parasites usually cause no major problem for the child.

1. How did my child contract this infection?

Pin worms are usually contracted by being passed on from one child to another. Adults who are caregivers to children can also become infected. The process occurs when a child ingests the eggs that are usually on his or her hands, having been transferred from someone else and subsequently ending up in the child's mouth. The eggs are then swallowed and transformed in the intestines through a life cycle process to the worm stage. These worms are often seen on the skin surrounding the child's anus, which is the site where the female worm migrates to lay the eggs. The process can start all over again if these eggs are later ingested by the child. The worms are usually whitish in color and measure from approximately 1/8 inch to 1/2 inch in length. The eggs can also be transmitted from bedding, bathtubs, toilet seats, and stuffed animals, as they can survive up to two to three days outside of the body.

2. Is it serious, and what are the symptoms associated with this condition?

Most children have no symptoms except for an itchy sensation around the anus. This symptom can keep a child up at night. Some children have minor abdominal discomfort. Others sometime develop a secondary bacterial infection in the area around the anus where the pin worms have irritated the skin. Rarely, in girls, the pin worms can crawl into the vagina and cause irritation. Also, there have been rare reports of the worms causing inflammation of the ovarian tubes and the urethra. Recurrent infections are very common and a child may reinfect him or herself by scratching the affected area and then putting hands in mouth.

3. What tests can be done to diagnose this condition?

At times the worms can be seen with the naked eye, most often in the area around the anus. This is sufficient evidence to make the diagnosis. Otherwise, one has to look for the eggs, which are microscopic in size. This is done by taking the sticky side of clear cellophane tape and dabbing the skin around the anus in several different areas. Then the tape is placed on a slide and the slide is examined under a microscope in the doctor's lab to see if eggs are present.

4. How is this condition treated?

Pin worm infections are treated with mebendazole, pyrantel pamoate, or albendazole, all of which are given in a single dose regimen and usually repeated in two weeks. Mebendazole is, by far, the most often prescribed medicine for this condition as it comes in a chewable tablet and the dose is one tablet for children and adults alike. All family members and close contacts should be treated as well, especially if the child has repeated infections. Scrupulous cleansing of the nails, bedding, night clothes, bathtub, and stuffed animals are essential. Washing hands before eating and avoiding nail biting should be included in the overall treatment regimen, as reinfection is very common. Some children contract pin worm infections repeatedly, and subsequent flare-ups should be treated in a similar manner as the initial infection.

5. What kind of follow-up is needed?

No follow-up is necessary if the treatment plan is carried out correctly and the child's symptoms disappear.

GREGORY R. ISTRE, M.D.
Infectious Diseases

PITYRIASIS ROSEA

Definition: A condition of the skin characterized by the sudden appearence of dry round or oval pink-brown spots, usually on the back, chest, arms, and thighs.

Author's Comment: This is an unattractive skin condition that fortunately goes away on its own with no specific treatment.

1. What causes this condition, and how did my child contract it?

Pityriasis rosea is a rash due to a viral infection. The virus is passed from person to person.

2. Is it contagious, and how is it spread?

The virus that started the rash is contagious, but the skin lesions themselves are not.

3. What is the natural course of this disease?

The rash often starts with a single, larger, red, scaly spot that can look a lot like ringworm. Mild cold symptoms, tiredness, or low-grade fever may also be noted prior to the rash. After a few days to a week, the child breaks out with many pink to pink-brown scaly spots, mostly on the chest, belly, and back, with less on the arms, legs, and neck. The skin lesions generally last six to eight weeks, then go away on their own.

4. Will the lesions move to the face?

The face is usually not affected, but a few spots can appear on neck and lower cheeks.

5. How is it treated?

There is no medication to make this rash go away, but sun exposure (without sun burning) can help skin lesions fade faster. If itching is present and bothersome, then antihistamines or anti-itch creams can give some relief.

6. Are there any potential side effects from the treatment?

Antihistamines can cause drowsiness. Anti-itch creams may cause skin irritation. Sun exposure should not be excessive and sunburns should be avoided.

7. How long will it take for the lesions to disappear?

Skin lesions typically clear in six to eight weeks. After the scaly lesions resolve, dark or light spots (discoloration) may be left behind; these will fade slowly over several months.

8. Under what conditions do I call you back?

Call back if the rash changes significantly, if fever develops, or if your child feels or acts sick. Most people with pityriasis rosea feel fine, except for the rash. You should also call back if skin lesions are noted on the palms of the hands.

9. When do you wish to see my child again for a follow-up?

Follow-up is needed if the rash is not much improved after six to eight weeks or if the rash worsens rather than improves.

K. ROBIN CARDER, MD
Dermatology

PNEUMONIA

Definition: Infection of the lungs.

Author's Comment: This condition can be a serious problem. However, assuming the child has a normal immune system, most children with close medical supervision and appropriate antibiotic therapy recover completely within one to two weeks. Keep in close communication with the doctor and be sure to return for follow-up exams.

1. What causes this condition, and how did my child contract it?

Pneumonia is an infection of the lungs. It is usually caused by germs, such as bacteria or viruses. Viral infections are the most common. Other causes include aspiration of food or other foreign substances and ingestion of hydrocarbons (e.g. petroleum products).

2. What are the dangers associated with this condition?

With early aggressive and appropriate antibiotic therapy for bacterial pneumonia, complications are few, and most children's recovery begins shortly after antibiotics are instituted. However, the child with pneumonia has to be followed closely to make sure that he or she is getting better. If the child is not drinking fluids adequately, if the oxygen saturation of the blood as determined in the doctor's office is at a dangerously low level, or if the child's respiratory condition appears to be getting worse, your pediatrician may elect to hospitalize him or her. By doing this, intravenous fluids, intravenous antibiotics, and more aggressive therapy with closer medical supervision can be given.

3. Is it contagious and, if so, for how long?

The bacteria or virus causing the pneumonia is contagious. An infected person spreads the germs through coughing, sneezing, and so on. If the pneumonia is caused by bacteria, the child is usually contagious until he or she has been on antibiotics for one to two days. If it is caused by a virus, then the contagious period usually persists until the child is clinically improved and free of fever.

4. Is there a need to obtain a chest X ray?

A chest X ray is definitive proof of having pneumonia. Sometimes the physical exam is strongly consistent with having pneumonia and the doctor may not order a chest X ray. If pneumonia occurs more than once, then a chest X ray should be obtained to substantiate the diagnosis.

5. What medicines are used to treat the condition?

Pneumonia caused by bacteria is treated with antibiotics. Circumstances associated with the pneumonia usually determine which antibiotics are used. This includes illness occurring in the hospital, outside of the hospital, and any preexisting or coexisting medical conditions. The full course of medication should be taken and not stopped early even if the child feels better.

Pneumonia caused by a virus will not respond to routine antibiotics. Supportive treatment includes getting adequate rest, fluids, and fever and cough medications.

6. What are the potential side effects of the medicines?

Any antibiotic has the potential to alter the normal healthy germs of the digestive system. If this occurs, then the person may get diarrhea. An allergic reaction to an antibiotic is another potential side effect.

7. Once medicines are started, how long will it take for my child to show signs of improvement?

In most situations, children begin to feel better within two full days on antibiotics. If symptoms do not improve or if they worsen, then the doctor should be contacted to reevaluate the child.

8. What should I look for that might indicate that the condition is getting worse?

Persistence or worsening of fever, cough, labored breathing, or shortness of breath may indicate that the pneumonia is worsening.

9. Under what conditions should I call you back?

You should always let the doctor's office know how your child is responding to treatment after two to three days, even if your child is improving. It is important for the doctor to know that the treatment plan is working. If there are any indications that the child is worsening, then the doctor should be called at that time.

10. When can my child resume activities and return to school?

Most children feel better within two to three days. They should be able to resume activities within four to seven days. When fever has resolved and the cough is no longer disruptive, then the child may return to school.

11. When do you wish to see my child again concerning this condition?

If the child's symptoms are not improving or if they are worsening, then he or she should be reexamined immediately. If the child is responding to treatment appropriately, then he or she should be rechecked within a month. The doctor will determine when the child should be reevaluated based on the assessment of the symptoms and clinical picture at the time of diagnosis.

RICHARD B. SILVER, MD
Pulmonary

POISON IVY

Definition: A type of dermatitis (skin rash) that originates from contact with a certain type of plant that has three leaves.

Author's Comment: Some children contract this condition over and over again and require rounds of treatment every time. There is still no vaccine to prevent poison ivy. The best advice I can give is find out where the poison ivy plant is and keep your child away from it.

1. How did my child contract poison ivy?
Poison ivy is contracted by contact with the resin from poison ivy, poison sumac, or poison oak plants.

2. How is it treated?
Topical or oral steroids are used to treat the skin inflammation, swelling, and itching. Oral steroids should be given for a minimum of two weeks to prevent the rebound worsening that occurs with shorter courses. Calamine lotion will soothe irritated skin. If the skin is blistered, weepy, and draining, then compresses with over-the-counter

Burrow's or Domeboro solution one to two times a day help to dry up the lesions. Washing the plant resin off of the skin and clothes is necessary to prevent further contact with other areas of skin.

3. What, if any, are the side effects of the treatment?

The most common side effects seen with short courses of oral steroids are increased appetite, mood changes, and irritability.

4. When can I expect the symptoms to improve and the rash to disappear?

Improvement of the itching is usually noted within two to three days, but it may take two to three weeks for the skin lesions to dry up completely. Some residual redness or dark discoloration of the skin may last for weeks to a few months but will fade gradually.

5. Can it spread from person to person?

If the plant resin remains on the skin or clothing (or on the fur of a pet) contact with the resin can spread the rash.

6. Will the clothes and linen that touch my child's skin need to be washed?

Yes. Anything that touched the plant (hands, face, clothing, gloves, coat sleeves) should be washed thoroughly.

7. What can be done to prevent it from occurring again?

Identifying the plant and having it removed from the yard is the best way to prevent future poison ivy rashes. Wearing long sleeves and gloves while doing yard work helps to limit contact with the plant.

There are also over-the-counter barrier lotions designed to protect the skin from direct plant contact. These need to be applied to the skin prior to any potential exposure (i.e., before going outside to do yard work). If clothes or hands have touched the plant, then the clothes should be removed carefully and placed in the washing machine, and the hands, face, and other areas of uncovered skin should be washed immediately and thoroughly.

8. Will there be any residual scarring?

Temporary discoloration of the skin is common, but permanent scarring is not typical. Scarring may occur if the reaction was very severe or if deep fingernail scratches injured the skin.

9. When can my child return to normal activities?

As soon as any swelling has gone down and your child feels up to it, he or she may return to normal activities.

10. What kind of follow-up is needed?

For more severe reactions involving the face, follow-up in a few days or a week may be needed. For milder cases, no follow-up is needed unless the rash returns or medication-related problems arise.

K. ROBIN CARDER, MD
Dermatology

PRECOCIOUS PUBERTY

Definition: A child showing early bodily signs of
               sexual development.

Author's Comment: The appearance of early bodily signs of sexual maturation is often a concern to both parents and doctors and needs to be investigated.

1. What causes this condition to exist in my child?

Enlargement of the breasts in girls or enlargement of the testes in boys can signify that the brain has triggered puberty to start. If these changes occur before age eight in girls or nine in boys, then they are classified as precocious. In girls, most of the time the cause is unknown but may be associated with any brain abnormality, from as mild as a previous concussion or as significant as a brain tumor. In boys, there is usually an explanation for this condition, and it may be a symptom of a serious medical problem.

Early appearance of pubic hair or underarm hair is caused by early activation of the adrenal glands. This may either be due to a benign cause and unassociated with other signs of puberty or may signify a congenital abnormality in hormone formation in the adrenal gland or adrenal tumor.

Occasionally, sexual development can be caused by a child's inadvertent exposure to hormone-containing compounds, such as ingestion of oral contraceptives or touching a parent who has used estrogen or testosterone creams or gels.

2. What are the long-term dangers that it poses?

There are really two considerations here. First, one must consider precocious puberty as a symptom, not a disease. As such, the question is whether it signifies the presence of an underlying disorder that could pose a health risk to the child. Certainly, in the case of a tumor or congenital abnormality in hormone synthesis, the risk is not of the puberty itself but of the disorder that has caused it.

Once such a disorder has been excluded, the risk of puberty itself could be considered. If puberty progresses too soon or too rapidly, a child is at risk of stopping growing prematurely and could become a very short adult. In addition, there may be some social stress to appearing much older than one's peer group.

3. What tests are needed to further evaluate this condition?

A visit with the pediatrician is crucial so that the timing and tempo of the pubertal changes can be evaluated. A bone age X ray of the hand may be performed to assess for the physical maturation of the skeleton; maturation is accelerated with exposure to either endogenous (internal) or exogenous (environmental) sex hormones. Blood tests may be performed to measure the levels of hormones generated by the pituitary gland, the ovaries or testes, or by the adrenal glands.

A pelvic ultrasound may be used to assess the internal maturity of the uterus and ovaries or evaluate for any tumors. A brain MRI may also be used to look for any anatomical abnormalities in the brain.

4. Do we need to see an endocrinologist (hormone specialist)?

Pediatric endocrinologists are pediatricians who have spent several extra years in training to learn about hormone disorders in children. Therefore, they are a valuable resource to you and your pediatrician in helping to define and manage a child with precocious puberty.

5. If the test proves there is something wrong, what is the treatment and how successful is it?

Again, there are several considerations here. If the cause is premature activation of the pituitary gland, medication can be administered to quiet the activity. Most of the time, an intramuscular injection is given every four weeks to suppress the activity. Any underlying abnormality of the brain, which may have caused the precocious puberty, would also need to be evaluated and, if possible, treated.

A congenital abnormality of hormone formation in the adrenal gland can be treated with oral medication that replaces the hormone that is not being produced and, in turn, would inhibit overproduction of the sex hormones.

Obviously any inadvertent exposures should be sought and eliminated, but if they have continued for a long duration, they may have triggered true activation of the pituitary gland.

Many girls who have slowly progressive signs of maturation one to two years early and have no significant disease as the cause require no specific treatment.

6. What kind of follow-up is needed for this condition, and when do you want to see my child again?

Again, because this category describes a multitude of conditions, the follow-up schedule can vary. Obviously, inadvertent exposures involve far fewer follow-ups than brain tumors. The follow-up would need to be specifically tailored to the individual child.

ELLEN S. SHER, MD
Endocrinology

PSORIASIS

Definition: A chronic, noncontagious skin disease characterized by red patches covered by thick white scale.

Author's Comment: This condition is more common than we would like to think. Most cases are mild but some are severe and can be quite disfiguring. The latter type is more likely to be treated by a dermatologist (skin specialist).

1. What causes this condition, and how did my child contract it?

Psoriasis is a condition that causes the skin to turn over at a faster rate than normal, leading to a buildup of scale on the skin. In some cases psoriasis can be inherited. It can also occur randomly and affect only one person in a family. The cause of psoriasis is unknown. In children, psoriasis may be triggered by strep infections of the skin or throat. Psoriasis is not contagious.

2. What is the natural course of this disorder?

In general, psoriasis is a chronic (long-term) skin condition for which we have no permanent cure. The skin lesions come and go. Because this condition improves with sun exposure, most people have milder disease in the summer, which worsens in the winter.

3. What is the treatment, and are there any potential side effects?

There are several ways to treat psoriasis. Topical treatment is usually started first unless the psoriasis is severe. Topical steroids are very useful in decreasing the redness, itch, and inflammation. They also help to make skin lesions less scaly and thick. Steroid creams are quite safe when used properly, but they can cause thinning of the skin if applied more often than directed or to normal (unaffected) skin for prolonged periods of time. Thinning of the skin can also occur if a potent steroid is used on delicate areas of skin (face, neck, groin, underarms), so it is important to follow your doctor's instructions closely and use the medications only as prescribed.

Vitamin D (calcipotriene) and vitamin A (tazarotene) topical creams are also effective in treating psoriasis and work nicely in combination with topical steroids. The most common side effect of these medications is skin irritation. If calcipotriene is used on large areas of the body in very young children, the blood calcium levels may increase, so occasional blood testing may be needed.

Tar and salicylic acid products have been used for a long time to treat psoriasis. Tar is very effective. It is available as a shampoo, cream, ointment, or a liquid to add to the bath. It is usually well tolerated but can be a little messy and may leave yellow-brown discoloration when used in the bathtub or on blonde hair. Some of the newer tar products are more elegant and less messy. Salicylic acid helps to decrease scaling and can be compounded into an ointment form for use on the skin. It is also used in scalp treatments and medicated shampoos for use on scalp psoriasis. Salicylic acid and tar work well in combination.

For more severe disease, there are oral medications that can be prescribed. These medications can affect the liver or kidneys, so bloodwork and regular follow-up to monitor side effects and progress are required. There is a new group of medications called "biologics" that seem promising, but at present there are very few studies evaluating their safety for use in children with psoriasis. These medications are given as injections or through an IV, and bloodwork is necessary.

4. Does ultraviolet light help, and, if so, is it safe for children?

Ultraviolet (UV) light is very helpful for psoriasis. UV light therapy is available in many dermatologists' offices. Brief sessions two to three times a week are needed for the treatment to be effective. The UV light exposure time is started low, then increased gradually so that burning does not occur. Natural sunlight can also be effective, but sunscreen should be worn and sunburns should be avoided. Use of tanning beds is not recommended for children.

5. What complications can occur as a result of this disorder?

Complications include psoriatic arthritis. Skin infections may occur at sites of scratches or open skin. Another complication is pustular psoriasis in which the skin worsens suddenly and becomes covered with pus-filled blisters. This can be a serious condition. It tends to occur after treatment with injected or oral steroids, so these treatments are not recommended for psoriasis treatment in children.

6. Will there be any personal disfigurement?

The scaly skin of psoriasis causes much embarrassment, especially for children and teenagers. Children with psoriasis often wear pants and long sleeves to hide their skin. Nevertheless, psoriasis lesions do not cause permanent scarring, and, with proper treatment, the skin can look normal.

7. Is there a specialist we need to see for this condition?

Psoriasis management can be challenging, so evaluation by a dermatologist is recommended. If your child has painful or swollen joints, then consultation with a rheumatologist (joint specialist) may also be needed.

8. When should I call you back?

If your child has strep throat (a known trigger of psoriasis), sudden worsening of his or her psoriasis (especially if pus bumps are present), signs of a skin infection, or is no longer responding to his or her medications, then you should call your doctor. You should also call if you think your child develops side effects or severe irritation from their medication.

9. When do you wish to see my child again concerning this condition?

After starting a new treatment, a follow-up visit in four to six weeks is recommended. Once on a good routine, follow-up visits only a few times a year may be all that is needed. More frequent visits may be needed if your child is taking an oral, intravenous, or injected medication.

K. ROBIN CARDER, MD
Dermatology

PYLORIC STENOSIS

Definition: An enlargement and tightening of the muscle in the lower stomach leading to obstruction with forceful vomiting.

Author's Comment: This condition of projectile vomiting in infancy is quite frightening for young parents. Actually, the required surgery to correct this condition, barring any unforeseen complications, is a very simple procedure by a competent pediatric surgeon, and the recovery time is short.

1. What causes this condition, and how did my child develop it?

Pyloric stenosis is a condition in which the pyloric valve at the end of the stomach thickens excessively and blocks off the connection (the pyloric channel) between the stomach and the first part of the intestine (duodenum). Food that the baby eats cannot pass from the stomach into the intestine. As a result, when the stomach contracts to try to push food into the duodenum, the baby vomits (usually forcefully). This condition typically occurs between three weeks to three months of age but can be seen within three days of birth up to rarely as old as nine months of age.

2. What are the potential complications that can occur from this disorder?

Dehydration occurs over the first few days followed by weight loss, severe salt imbalance, lethargy, and death.

3. What tests are needed to substantiate the diagnosis?

A history of progressively worsening "projectile" vomiting after feeds, dehydration and physical exam demonstrating a palpable enlarged pyloric muscle frequently point to the diagnosis. However, many children develop the symptoms slowly (over one to two weeks) and are frequently diagnosed with formula intolerance or gastroesophageal acid reflux. In any instance, an abdominal ultrasound will typically demonstrate an enlarged pylorus. Barium studies can also demonstrate pyloric stenosis, though abdominal ultrasound is the preferred study.

4. What is the standard treatment of this disorder?

The standard care involves stabilization of the child's condition by correcting dehydration and the child's electrolyte (salt) imbalance. This may take several hours to several days depending on how ill the child is when diagnosed.

After the child has been stabilized, surgery is performed to open up the pyloric channel. Most surgeons perform a pyloromyotomy in which the pyloric muscle is cut. This relaxes the muscle and opens up the inside of the channel. This operation can be done as a standard "open" procedure (using an incision) and as laparoscopic procedures (using a camera placed through the belly button and two tiny incisions).

5. What are the potential complications of the treatment?

Complications are rare but include the following:

- Internal bleeding
- Injury to the stomach or intestine with leakage of stomach contents into the abdominal cavity
- Incomplete cutting of the muscle, resulting in continued symptoms
- Wound infection

6. Will there be any residual problems following the proposed treatment?

Unless there is a complication, residual problems are rare. If the muscle is not completely cut, the child will exhibit continued symptoms.

7. What if nothing is done—is there a chance that this condition will resolve on its own?

Pyloric stenosis can resolve, but it requires many months in the hospital with intravenous feeding or attempted passage of a feeding tube past the obstructing pyloric muscle. Children treated surgically are typically in the hospital for one to four days with a lower complication rate. Nonoperative management of pyloric stenosis is not recommended.

8. What kind of follow-up is needed?

Usually, your surgeon will want to see your child two to three weeks after surgery to make sure that everything is going well. After that, any follow-up is rarely necessary.

KEVIN M. KADESKY, MD
Surgery

RHEUMATOID ARTHRITIS–JUVENILE

Definition: A condition characterized by chronic
inflammation of the joints and
surrounding tissue leading, at times, to
chronic deformities.

Author's Comment: This condition can cause much discomfort and pain during childhood and, in severe cases, can lead to chronic disability. It requires that the family work closely with the doctor to establish a treatment regimen that works.

1. What causes this condition, and how did my child contract it?

No one for sure truly knows what causes this condition. Some forms of rheumatism seem to occur after a viral infection or bacterial infection, especially strep. These types of rheumatism are often self-limiting, meaning they occur for a period of time, up to six months, and typically go away. These are known as postreactive arthritis or postreactive rheumatism. True juvenile rheumatoid arthritis (JRA) occurs for no known reason at this time.

2. Is it genetic?

In some cases, rheumatism certainly seems to run in the family. There are some genetic predispositions toward it, and there are some genetic markers that are seen more commonly in people with forms of rheumatoid arthritis, but there is no clear-cut gene that causes rheumatoid arthritis. However, there is some thought that certain genes may increase one's risk of rheumatoid arthritis.

3. What are the complications that can occur as a result of this condition?

There are many complications that can occur. In terms of the joints themselves, pain, stiffness, deformities, and, sometimes, painful and disabling arthritis requiring surgery can occur. However, this is uncommon in most forms of JRA. Other complications can occur in other body parts. JRA can affect the eyes, and it is important to have the child's eyes checked at least once a year. Permanent problems with vision can develop if undetected and untreated over many years. Some forms of rheumatism can affect other body parts, such as the heart, lungs, kidneys, and even the nervous system; these are rare complications, but they can occur. It is important to follow up with a pediatric rheumatologist.

4. What treatment can be used?

Currently there are a number of treatment options available. For mild forms of childhood rheumatism, an anti-inflammatory medication can be tried, such as naproxen. For a lot of children with mild forms of JRA, this is sufficient. Giving an over-the-counter medication, such as naproxen, over months can cause injury to the kidneys or liver or cause blood pressure problems. Therefore, monitoring is important.

There are other medications that can be used that suppress the immune system and, in so doing, suppress the rheumatoid arthritis. However, these have much more potential side effects and need to be carefully weighed with the guidance of a rheumatologist, especially with use of methotrexate and cyclophosphamide.

5. Are there any potential side effects from the treatment?

Use of anti-inflammatories over many years can cause damage to the kidneys, formation of ulcers, high blood pressure, or liver damage. Methotrexate and cyclophosphamide have much more serious complications. They suppress the immune system and increase the risk of infection. Furthermore, these medications can affect the bone marrow, cause anemia, cause osteoporosis, and can interact with many other medications (even over-the-counter medications). It is important to be aware of all medications the child is taking. Any new medication should be discussed with the rheumatologist, pediatrician, and/or pharmacist.

6. What criteria do we use to judge if the treatment is working?

The child's level of comfort and/or swelling, the child's physical response, and the blood work are all taken into consideration. With some forms of rheumatism, however, the blood work will be persistently abnormal, yet the child's symptoms might improve. The biggest marker of whether the treatment is working is the child's response, and the blood work is the next marker.

7. Is there anything we can do to prevent long-term complications from this disorder?

An important step is to maintain joint flexibility and strength, as well as maintain good nutrition. Often seeing a physical therapist for gentle exercise instruction is important. If the arthritis is severely affecting weight-bearing joints, such as the hips, knees, and ankles, then learning to do activities that strengthen the joints without putting excessive force on them is important; the most common exercises are bicycling, swimming, or simple walking. It is also important to teach children about what rheumatism means for them in terms of their level of activity.

8. Do we need to see a rheumatologist (arthritis specialist)?

Typically, your pediatrician is the person best trained to see initially with this problem, but a referral to a pediatric rheumatologist is likely. Rheumatism does not just affect the joints, but it can affect the soft tissues and can cause various body parts to be affected in various ways. Sometimes it can be difficult to determine if another problem is an effect of the rheumatism or of a truly different disease. A rheumatologist is skilled in sorting out these types of problems.

9. What circumstances would require me to call you concerning my child's condition?

One of the biggest concerns would be that of infection. If the child develops a high fever for no good reason, suddenly develops increased swelling in a joint, or develops a sudden inability to walk, these could be markers for an infection. Infection can occur in joints that are already involved with rheumatoid arthritis. If the child begins to vomit blood or pass blood in the stools as a complication of anti-inflammatory medication, this can mean that ulcers are developing.

10. When do you wish to see my child again regarding this disorder?

Typically the child should be followed based on age in terms of wellness visits and immunizations as recommended. There is no specific schedule to follow the child for the rheumatoid arthritis over and above what the rheumatologist might recommend. There are very few pediatric rheumatologists in this country, and there can be large geographic distance between the rheumatologists. As a result the pediatrician can act as the intermediary between the child and the rheumatologist, discussing observations, blood draws, and laboratory analyses.

W. BARRY HUMENIUK, MD
Orthopedics

RINGWORM OF BODY
(Tinea Corporis)

Definition: A fungal infection of the skin on the body.

Author's Comment: This condition can be easily treated. The word "ringworm" refers to the round lesion with the elevated (ring-like) border, not an actual worm. You may have to be a good detective to find out how your child contracted this skin infection.

1. What is the cause of this condition, and how did my child contract it?

Ringworm is a very common fungal infection of the skin and can occur at any age. It is usually due to contact with an infected person or animal (such as a stray cat). Contact with infected children at school or daycare is the most common way to contract ringworm, but sometimes it is difficult to pinpoint the exact source of your child's infection.

2. Is it contagious and, if so, for how long?

Yes, it is contagious if others come in direct contact with the skin lesions. Once treated, they are no longer contagious.

3. Do we need to contact the people with whom my child has been in contact?

If your child has been in direct physical contact with others (either in the classroom or on a sports team), it is a good idea to notify those individuals, as well as their parents, teachers, and coaches, so that they can be treated early if they become infected.

4. How is it treated?

For ringworm on the skin, topical antifungal medications applied two to three times daily for about two to four weeks (until the lesions have cleared completely) is usually sufficient. If steroid creams, such as hydrocortisone, have been used on the lesions previously or if the lesions involve areas of longer hair growth, such as the eyebrows or scalp, then oral antifungal medication is required. Creams combining a topical steroid with an antifungal medication are not recommended for ringworm and can delay clearing of the infection.

5. What are the potential side effects of the treatment?

The creams are usually well tolerated but may be irritating if applied to open or cracked skin. Oral antifungal medications can interact with other medications and may affect the liver, so these medications should be monitored by a physician familiar with their uses and should be used with caution in people with liver disease.

6. How long will it take to clear up?

Ringworm will usually clear up after two to four weeks of topical therapy or one to four weeks of oral therapy. The infection will take longer to clear up if areas of longer hair growth are involved or if a topical steroid has been used on the skin lesions previously.

7. How do we prevent this condition from coming back?

The best way to keep lesions from coming back is to identify and treat the source of infection (usually another child or a pet). Skin lesions should be treated until they have completely cleared. Also, any other family members with signs of ringworm should be treated so that the infection does not continue to be passed from one family member to another.

8. Do we need to see a dermatologist?

If the infection is not improving after two to four weeks, if oral treatment is needed, or if the diagnosis is not certain, then your child may need to see a dermatologist.

9. When do you wish to see my child again for this condition?

If the skin lesions are clearing up with treatment, no follow-up may be needed unless the rash returns. But, if the infection has been prolonged or if your child requires oral medication, then a follow-up visit two to four weeks after starting treatment may be needed.

K. ROBIN CARDER, MD
Dermatology

RINGWORM OF SCALP
(Tinea Capitis)

Definition: Fungal infection of the scalp.

Author's Comment: This condition needs to be treated with oral medication. Creams by themselves will not clear it up. Fortunately, you do not have to shave your child's head and have him or her wear a beanie like they did in the old days.

1. What is the cause of this condition, and how did my child contract it?

Ringworm of the scalp is a fungal infection that involves not only the skin but also the hair follicles. In most cases, ringworm is spread from one child to another, but occasionally it can be contracted from a pet (usually a new or stray cat).

2. Are there any tests that need to be done to better establish the cause?

Some cases are obvious and require no testing. Nevertheless, there are other scalp conditions that resemble ringworm, so a fungal culture of the hair is usually recommended to verify that the child has ringworm. Also, hair can also be examined under the microscope to look for fungus. Because several months of oral medication are required to treat ringworm, you want to be sure of the diagnosis before you start treatment, so testing is recommended if the diagnosis of ringworm is uncertain.

3. What should we do to find the source?

The most common sources are other children, siblings, and pets. Start by looking at the scalps of your other children to see if they have any signs of ringworm. Examine your pets for signs of hair loss or scaly skin, and ask your child if he or she played with any pets or stray animals prior to the infection. Next, notify your child's school or daycare teacher that your child has ringworm and ask if anyone else in the class has had ringworm. Finding the source is not always easy, since some children are ringworm "carriers" and may lack scalp lesions or obvious signs of infection.

4. Is it contagious and, if so, for how long?

Yes. Ringworm is contagious until treated. Interestingly, most children pick up ringworm from asymptomatic carriers (children who have fungus on their scalp but show no signs of it). Therefore, the old practice of keeping children with obvious infections out of school is not that helpful, since the carriers who are difficult to detect remain in the classroom. Using selenium sulfide or ketoconazole shampoo to wash the scalp twice weekly helps to decrease contagiousness; it can also prevent uninfected children from getting the infection.

5. Do we need to contact the people with whom my child has been in contact?

Yes. Classmates, teachers, coaches of sports teams, and hairdressers in contact with your child should be notified.

6. Does my child need to wear a cap or any other type of head covering?

This is not necessary. Using a selenium sulfide or ketoconazole shampoo twice weekly is prevention enough. If you feel better having your child wear a head covering or cap, be sure to wash it regularly so that fungus does not remain on the cap and cause reinfection of the scalp. Caution should also be used not to share hats, hairbrushes, or combs with others.

7. What medication should be taken to treat this disorder and for how long?

Oral medication is needed to cure ringworm. Griseofulvin, terbinafine, or itraconazole are the most commonly used medications for scalp ringworm. Treatment for two to four months is often required. Medication should be continued for two weeks after the last scalp lesion clears up, or until a repeat fungal culture is negative. Because oral antifungals can affect the liver, bloodwork (labs) may be required for terbinafine or itraconazole therapy but is generally not necessary for griseofulvin unless your child has a history of liver disease or is taking other medications that interact with this drug. It should be noted that terbinafine is less effective for the type of ringworm that comes from animals. The effectiveness of griseofulvin improves if the medication is taken with fatty foods, such as milk or cheese. Itraconazole is best taken with something acidic, such as a soda.

8. Will the medicine cure the disease?

Yes. Therapy with an appropriate antifungal for a sufficient period of time is curative. Reinfection may occur if treatment is stopped too early. Repeating a fungal culture at the end of therapy to be sure the infection has cleared can prevent this. Reinfection can also occur if the child comes back into contact with an infected pet or child.

9. Are there any potential side effects from the medication?

Oral antifungal medications can interact with some other medications and may affect the liver, so these medications should be monitored by a physician familiar with their use and should be avoided in people with significant liver disease. Some oral antifungals should also be used with caution if your child has a heart arrhythmia (irregularity in heart rhythm). Drug rashes or allergic reactions to these medications may also occur but are uncommon.

10. When do we expect to see improvement?

Some improvement (decreased redness, scaling, itching, or tenderness) can usually be noted after two to three weeks of treatment, but it usually takes at six to eight weeks for hair to start growing back.

11. Do we need to see a dermatologist?

If the diagnosis is uncertain, if the infection is severe, or if your child is not improving as expected with proper oral treatment, then you may need to see a dermatologist.

12.   When do you wish to see my child again for this condition?

A follow-up visit four to six weeks after starting therapy is recommended to assure that the child is improving as expected. Lab work may also be required at this visit.

K. ROBIN CARDER, MD
Dermatology

ROSEOLA

Definition: Baby measles.

Author's Comment: This condition can be frightening for a parent, because of the four- to five-day high fever that the child experiences. The appearance of a rash at the end of the fever is almost a welcome relief, because it finally signifies to the doctor the true identity of the disease.

1. What causes this disease, and how did my child contract it?

Roseola is usually a mild disease caused by primary infection with human herpes virus (HHV) strains 6 or 7. This common infection generally occurs in children between the ages of three months to three years, and causes three to seven days of high fever. Some children may also develop swollen lymph nodes in the neck and head, runny nose, vomiting, or diarrhea. After the fever resolves, a rash may appear, starting on the trunk and abdomen and then spreading to the arms and neck. This rash may last several days. The virus is spread by direct contact with an infected person's saliva or respiratory secretions.

2. What is the natural course of the disease?

Children with this infection usually recover fully within a week of the onset of the fever.

3. Is it contagious and, if so, for how long?

Individuals with roseola are contagious until about one to two days after the fever has resolved.

4. When was my child first contagious?

Children are first contagious from about two days prior to the onset of the fever.

5. Are there any complications that can occur as a result of this disease?

In 10 percent to 15 percent of children with this infection, seizures can occur during the period of high fevers. Seek emergency care if your child has a seizure, but the fever-related seizures are usually short, self-resolved, and rarely harmful.

6. What is the treatment?

There is no specific treatment for roseola in persons with normal immune systems. Supportive care can be given to your child, with over-the-counter medications to reduce fever and oral fluids to prevent dehydration.

7. Should I notify people who have been in recent contact with my child, and, if so, what advice should be given?

Most individuals have already experienced infection by four years of age and have therefore developed immunity to HHV-6. Recent contacts of a child with roseola can be observed for the development of similar symptoms, which would occur after an incubation period of about ten days.

8. What limitations should be imposed on my child's activities during this illness?

A child with roseola should be kept at home and away from other children until the fever has been gone for one to two days. Family members of the ill child should wash their hands frequently to prevent the spread of these viruses to persons who may not be immune.

9. Can my child contract this again in the future?

Once a person has experienced infection and developed antibodies to the virus, he or she is immune to second infection. Following initial infection, the virus persists lifelong, usually asymptomatically but may reactivate to cause illness in persons with weakened immune systems.

10. What kind of follow-up is needed?

Unless there are complications, your child usually does not need to be seen again for this illness.

WENDY CHUNG, MD
Infectious Diseases

SCABIES

Definition: A skin disease caused by a mite and characterized by areas of inflammation on the skin and intense itching.

Author's Comment: This disease is sometimes difficult to recognize in a child and gets confused with other skin conditions. Once recognized, however, it can be adequately treated. Because it is contagious, the school needs to be informed so they can be on the lookout for other children with the same condition.

1. What causes this condition, and how did my child contract it?

Human scabies is a highly contagious skin disease caused by mites and is spread by direct skin contact with an infected person. In older children, the rash tends to involve the finger webs, wrists, groin, and under the arms. In infants, the rash often affects the face, scalp, palms, and soles.

2. What problems can be incurred as a result of scabies?

The rash caused by this skin mite is intensely itchy, especially at night.

3. What is the treatment, and how effective is it?

Application to the skin of permethrin 5 percent cream (Elimite) is over 90 percent effective as treatment for scabies. Oral antihistamines and topical steroids may help with itching. All family members and close contacts of the affected child should also be treated at the same time.

4. Are there any potential side effects of the treatment?

Other than some stinging, side effects of the medication are minimal.

5. How long will it take for the rash to clear up?

Relief from itching usually occurs within forty-eight hours of treatment. Despite effective treatment, skin nodules with some itching may remain for weeks.

6. How is it passed from one person to another, and how long will my child be contagious once appropriate treatment has begun?

Since the mite can survive for a few days off the human body, scabies can also be transmitted by contact with contaminated clothing and bedding. To prevent reinfection, all clothing, bedding, and towels should be washed with hot water. Items could also be placed in a sealed plastic bag for a week. Since transmission of mites is not likely more than twenty-four hours after treatment, children should be allowed to return to school or daycare after completion of treatment.

7. When do you wish to see my child again regarding this condition?

Most children do not need to be seen again after completing treatment. But if the itching continues for more than two weeks after treatment, the child should be reexamined for mites.

WENDY CHUNG, MD
Infectious Diseases

SCHOOL PHOBIA

Definition: **Fear of going to school.**

Author's Comment: This condition can cause much frustration and fear on the part of the parent. The family should work closely with the doctor and other recommended specialists to help get through this problem area.

1. What is causing my child to act in this manner?

School phobia is a specific subtype of separation anxiety disorders and is often caused by parental ambivalence or anxiety regarding a separation from their children. Parents will struggle to soothe their child when they are dealing with their own intense anxiety, and this continues to worsen the cycle of anxiety for that child until he or she begins refusing to go to school or to sleep alone. In some cases, school phobia could be an early sign of possible future development of generalized anxiety or socializing disorder.

2. Is there anything that I, as a parent, am doing that is affecting the situation adversely?

Parents can often, unwittingly, contribute to separation difficulties through their efforts to care for and to protect (or overprotect) their children. Examples would include allowing their child to sleep in their bed or to stay home when he or she begins to experience physical symptoms such as headaches or stomachaches. Often a parent will give in when a child throws a tantrum prior to or at the beginning of the school integration process.

3. Should I discuss the situation with the teachers and get them involved in the treatment program?

Yes, involvement of school officials and teachers can be key in helping a child overcome his or her school phobia early and get settled in the classroom. This allows the parents to leave the child behind and provides the necessary comfort during that separation. It is important that the process of dropping off children be brief and that it has been explained so that the children can already anticipate that early morning transition with the identified school official.

4. Are there any further diagnostic steps that need to be taken to uncover any possible underlying problems?

First and foremost, it is important to be sure that when the child complains of aches and pains, they are not legitimate physical problems. Often headaches or stomachaches will occur on the Sunday evening before school begins or during early morning routines in addition to the school setting.

5. What else can be done to make this situation better?

Often both parents have to be involved in the process of helping children overcome their school phobia. Many times one parent has inadvertently slipped into the "overprotective" mode and needs assistance in setting firm limits with his or her child.

6. Should we consult a psychologist or a psychiatrist?

A psychologist or psychiatrist should only be consulted if the problems persist or tend to escalate in spite of these behavioral interventions. A psychologist could certainly help to identify specific themes that may be occurring that are contributing to the school phobia. Examples would include conflicted family dynamics or the possibility that there is a legitimate stressor in the school causing the child's phobia (such as a bully or other negative peer or student–teacher interactions). A psychiatrist would be consulted if one is considering the possibility of a more significant anxiety or depressive disorder that may require medication intervention.

7. What kind of follow-up will be needed with you?

The pediatrician and/or psychologist/psychiatrist will likely set definite follow-up dates to help guide you and your child through this challenging period in your lives.

DANTE BURGOS, MD
Psychiatry

SCOLIOSIS

Definition: Curvature of the spine.

Author's Comment: This condition needs to be followed closely by your child's doctor or at a recommended orthopedic facility. Most children end up needing no treatment, but occasionally the condition will progress to the point where more aggressive therapy is needed.

1. What causes this condition to occur in my child?

Scoliosis occurs at different ages and for different potential reasons. The common version of scoliosis is the type that occurs in preadolescence to adolescence, mainly in girls, and has no currently known cause. There is a genetic component of scoliosis, but there is no identifiable gene or genetic test to determine if one is at risk for developing scoliosis, other than family history.

Other children with scoliosis are born with abnormalities of the spine, but this is very uncommon. Some children will develop scoliosis due to an abnormality of the spine development; this is also unusual as well, but it is looked for during the examination of the child. Other conditions that can cause scoliosis are underlying imbalances in the nervous or musculature system.

2. Is it hereditary?

The type of scoliosis that occurs in preadolescence and adolescence can be hereditary. If the family history is positive for scoliosis, the children should be screened. Other disorders that can cause scoliosis are abnormalities of the spinal cord or brain and are not typically hereditary.

3. What is the natural progression of this disorder?

The natural progression is unpredictable. Some people have scoliosis that never changes, some have scoliosis that progresses a little bit and then becomes static, some people have scoliosis that progresses and requires treatment. Once a curve starts to develop, it can progress at a rate of one degree every month. So, over the course of an entire year, a curve can progress twelve degrees. Rarely can it progress more; it is a very variable condition. An important feature is that it can progress while the child is still growing.

Once the child has completed growth and the skeleton is mature, as long as the curve is less than forty degrees, it will not progress as an adult. If the curve is greater than forty degrees, there is a steadily increasing risk that the curve will progress, even after the child has completed growth. The size of the curve at the end of growth is an important feature to note because this determines the lifetime risk of progression.

4. What symptoms can occur because of this condition?

Most scoliosis is completely asymptomatic and causes no pain or discomfort at all in the early stage. Since there are no early symptoms, the early diagnosis of scoliosis is made with screening.

Scoliosis is common enough now that school nurses screen for this, as well as the pediatrician upon a wellness examination at the age of six years and beyond.

Symptoms can occur because of scoliosis, the most common being the child holding one shoulder higher than the other or sometimes having a feeling of imbalance. Once the curve becomes larger than forty degrees, back pain can start to occur. When the spine curves to this degree, it puts abnormal forces on the joints of the back that can cause pain. Sometimes the ribs will literally bend over and touch the pelvic bone, which can cause discomfort. Curves that progress beyond sixty degrees can start to cause measurable changes in lung function. Curves that progress beyond eighty degrees can cause changes in heart function and become life threatening.

5. How will this condition limit my child's participation in athletics?

Scoliosis itself does not interfere with activities. Children or adults who have scoliosis can be active and do any activity. In fact, there are good reasons to be physically active to keep your child's muscles in balance and his or her posture well aligned. To that end, physical activity is encouraged. Participation in athletics is not limited by having scoliosis.

6. What is the treatment for this disorder?

The treatment depends on the degree of the curvature. Curves that are less than twenty degrees are just observed and checked periodically with repeat physical examinations and X rays. If the curve of the spine becomes larger than twenty degrees, the degree of maturity of the spine and pelvis are used to judge the risk or further progression.

Based on this knowledge, a decision for bracing may be recommended. In children who have a lot of growth remaining whose curves are larger than twenty degrees, bracing may well be recommended.

There are two options for bracing, either full time or nighttime. The Boston brace is the full-time brace, also referred to as TLSO. The Boston brace is considered full-time bracing and needs to be worn for at least eighteen hours a day. With some curves that affect only the lower back, there is an option for wearing a nighttime brace known as a Charleston brace; this is worn only during sleeping. There are only a few curves where this brace can be used.

Physical therapy has not been objectively shown to improve the condition, but it certainly helps from a sense of well-being and overall good health. I believe it is important to learn good back mechanics and posture. A short course of physical therapy to teach these behaviors is helpful. Along the same line, other activities that help teach posture, balance, and form, such as dance or martial arts, can also be helpful.

The next level of treatment is surgery. Surgery is reserved for children whose curves are progressing despite the use of a brace and whose curves are larger than forty degrees. The main reason for recommending scoliosis surgery is that curves that are larger than forty degrees are likely to continue to increase as time passes. In many respects the sooner that scoliosis surgery is accomplished to straighten the spine and keep it from curving, the easier it is technically to do the surgery. The surgery itself has a fairly lengthy recovery time; it takes almost three months to recover from having the spine straightened and fused. Scoliosis surgery can be done into the adult years, but with age, the spine is stiffer and the potential for difficulties and complications is greater.

The surgery itself involves straightening the spine and holding the spine straight with a series of metal rods placed into the spine to keep it straight while the bone fuses. The tradeoff is that it takes the spine that is flexible and curved and changes it to a spine that is straight, fused, and stiff. The decision to proceed with surgery does not need to be rushed. There is plenty of time to seek a second or third opinion. This is a major, potentially life-threatening surgery that involves a lot of blood loss and a long period of recovery. On average, it takes most people six weeks from the surgery date to feel comfortable again and almost three months to regain energy.

7. How often will X rays be required to follow its progress?

This depends on the age of the person upon diagnosis, the maturity of the spine, and the degree of curve. Since the fastest rate of progression of a curve is roughly one degree per month, most orthopedists will perform X rays every six months to follow curve progression. If rapid curve progression is suspected, the X rays can be requested every four months. Since X rays involve radiation, it is important to try and keep the X rays to those that are needed and not more.

Upon the initial diagnosis, it is important to get an X ray of the spine looking at it from the front and side. To just follow the scoliosis itself, a front view X ray only is needed; this cuts the radiation dose in half. Doing another X ray to take a look at the spine from the side really only needs to be done again if surgery is being contemplated for a final picture of the spine. X rays can be done to show the spine with shielding of important organs. In young females, the breasts can be shielded with special lead aprons. The gonads in males can also be shielded. If the X ray technician does not offer to do this, it is important to request this shielding.

8. Are there any exercises that can be performed to strengthen the back and to slow down the progression of this condition?

There are no studies on the value of exercise in slowing down scoliosis. Regardless of the condition, it is important to learn good back posture, training, and mechanics. To this end, seeing a physical therapist for some back exercises is useful. Other activities that are useful for controlling the back and helping alignment are yoga, dance, and martial arts.

9. What role does surgery play in the correction of this disorder?

Surgery plays the ultimate role in straightening the spine once the spine has curved more than forty degrees. Surgery straightens the spine and removes the curve. To keep the curve from coming back, the spine is straightened, metal rods are inserted, and the spine is fused. As a result, the spine is taken from a flexible curve to a rigid, straight spine. The results of spine surgery can result in mechanical problems of the back decades later. Further back surgery may be required.

10. Do we need to be referred to a doctor or institution that specializes in this condition?

Like any medical condition, one should see a physician and/or institution trained to take care of that particular disorder. Pediatric orthopedists are trained to take care of scoliosis. Only a small percentage of adult spine surgeons perform scoliosis surgery, and they treat the patients as adults, not young, growing people. There are some centers that specialize in scoliosis surgery only and some that treat a variety of orthopedic issues. If you have any questions regarding the physician's training or experience, please ask. The Internet is very useful tool in this regard as well.

11.   What kind of follow-up will be needed in the future?

The follow-up depends on the age of your child, the size of the curve, and the potential for curve progression. In general, scoliosis is followed until (1) the child completes growth and the curve does not require treatment or (2) the child continues to grow and the curve grows to the point of requiring treatment. Once the child's spine has completed growth, no further follow-up studies are needed. If scoliosis reaches the point of requiring surgery, once the spine has been fused there is a one-year follow-up. If there have been no complications after one year, no further follow-up is needed.

W. BARRY HUMENIUK, MD
Orthopedics

SEIZURES

Definition: Convulsions.

Author's Comment: These episodes are always very frightening. Fortunately, today there are newer medications available to treat the seizures that are quite effective when used by themselves or in combination with other medications under strict doctor's supervision. On the bright side, many children outgrow certain types of these convulsive disorders.

1. What causes this condition, and how did my child develop it?

A seizure is an episode that is the result of excessive activity of a group of nerve cells in the brain. There are different types of seizures. They may consist of staring, turning the body to one side, or jerking of the arms and legs either on one side or both sides. What type of seizure your child has is often dependent upon the cause for the seizure. Sometimes in young children (six months to five years of age), fever may cause a seizure, but not all seizures associated with fever in young children are due to the fever. Increasingly today, we are finding genetic causes that can result in seizures. Sometimes these are inherited, and sometimes they represent a new mutation in the child.

Abnormalities in the structure of the brain can also cause seizures. These abnormalities can be the result of the brain not forming properly, such as with focal cortical dysplasia or congenital malformations of the brain. Injury or trauma to the brain can cause scarring that can cause seizures. Infection, tumor, and stroke are also causes of seizures, although fortunately tumors and strokes in children are uncommon causes. Sometimes even a decreased blood flow to the brain, as can occur with a fainting episode, may result in a brief seizure.

2. Can the type of seizures that my child has cause brain damage?

It is possible that with very long seizures (greater than fifteen to thirty minutes) or with very frequent seizures, brain injury may occur. But in most cases, there is no evidence that brief seizures, especially when infrequent, cause brain damage.

3. What tests are needed to better establish the cause?

In many instances, if a child is taken to an emergency room following a seizure, he or she will have some blood and urine tests. If the child had previously been normal and healthy, these are usually normal. In most cases, the doctor will want to look at your child's brain with either a CT or MRI head scan. In most instances if your child has previously been normal and healthy and recovers from the seizure, an MRI head scan is the preferred way to look at your child's brain. Your doctor will also want to get a brain wave test (electroencephalogram). If your child has a fever, the doctor may want to do a spinal tap (lumbar puncture).

4. What medicines are used to control the seizures?

There are a number of medications available today to treat seizures. Decisions about which medication is best for your child may be dependent upon the type of seizure that your child has or the cause for the seizure. Some of the older medications used to treat seizures include phenobarbital, phenytoin (Dilantin), carbamazepine (Tegretol), and valproic acid (Depakote).

In the last fifteen years, a number of new medications have come onto the market. These include lamotrigine (Lamictal), topiramate (Topamax), levetiracetam (Keppra), gabapentin (Neurontin), and others. While these newer medications have not been shown to be more effective in treating seizures, in some instances they do offer safety advantages.

5. How long will my child need to stay on these medicines, and what are their potential side effects?

How long your child will be treated will depend on a number of factors including whether or not your child is completely seizure free on medication and the underlying cause for the seizures. In many instances, if a child's seizures are completely controlled for between two and four years, it is reasonable to give the child a trial off medication. About 65 percent of children will remain seizure free while 35 percent will relapse. Like any medication, there is always the potential of side effects. In general, these medications are quite safe.

The most common side effect is sleepiness. This will usually go away once the child gets used to the medication. Other side effects, such as dizziness, and behavioral problems can be seen. Other individual side effects may be seen with a particular medication, and your doctor will discuss that with you during the process of choosing what medication to use.

6. Do we need to consult with a neurologist?

In most cases, your pediatrician will want your child to see a neurologist. There may be rare instances, such as if a child has a brief seizure associated with fainting or if your child has a seizure clearly associated with a fever, where a neurological consultation is not necessary.

7. When do you wish to see my child again for this condition?

If a neurological consultation is not necessary, such as with a febrile seizure, a specific follow-up examination is not necessary. If your doctor decides that it would be best for your child to see a neurologist, then the neurologist will discuss follow-up with you.

ROY D. ELTERMAN, MD
Neurology

SEXUAL ABUSE
(Suspected)

Author's Comment: Sexual abuse of a child can range from inappropriate touching, fondling, or kissing of sexual organs to actual intercourse by either a stranger or person known to the child. If you suspect this very frightening event has occurred to your child, contact the doctor's office as soon as possible.

1. What agency do I contact to report my suspicions and to help me investigate the situation?

A suspicion of child sexual abuse should be reported to the local police department. Depending on the circumstances, Child Protective Services should be contacted as well. If you are unsure whether to report suspicions or who to call, discuss your concerns with your child's pediatrician. An alternative source of information available twenty-four hours a day is the National Child Abuse Hotline (800–422–4453/800–4–A–CHILD).

2. How do I go about investigating whether an incident truly took place?

The age of your child will determine how much information your child can give you. However, if you have a suspicion of sexual abuse, contact your doctor or your local police department. If you suspect recent or ongoing abuse, it is important to report your suspicions as quickly as possible. Ultimately, the job of investigating a potential incident will be the responsibility of the local authorities and not yours as the parent.

3. What type of proof do I need?

In cases of sexual abuse, tangible proof may be difficult to obtain. Sometimes there will be evidence of abuse found on physical exam. However, proof is not needed to warrant an investigation. If you suspect sexual abuse, contact your doctor or the police department immediately, whether or not you have proof.

4. Do I need to remove my child from the suspicious environment?

If there is a question of sexual abuse, it is best to remove your child from the suspicious environment. Trust your instincts. Children have limited means to protect themselves. Removing your child from any potential further harm is the safest alternative.

5. Should my child be seen by any specific medical facility that would more legally substantiate my accusations or suspicions?

Your child's pediatrician is a good place to start for direction on where to go for further evaluation if needed. In some cases a physical exam could provide forensic evidence for prosecution of the abuser. The earlier the exam is done relative to the suspected abuse, the greater the chance for obtaining forensic evidence. However, physical evidence is only found in a small percentage of exams.

There are strict criteria for maintaining the chain of custody of evidence in rape or sexual abuse cases. This type of exam should be done by doctors who are experienced in pediatric sexual assault and the procedures for maintaining evidence. The exam is performed in a way that is as gentle and as noninvasive as possible. In some cases, an exam is required to treat injuries, evaluate for possible internal injuries, or to test for sexually transmitted infections. If the victim is a girl who has begun to go through puberty, medication to prevent pregnancy may be offered.

6. Should I have my child seen by a therapist to counteract any possible psychological damage?

Even without physical injury, sexual abuse can result in psychological damage with long-lasting effects. This can be true whether the abuse was a one-time event or a series of events over time. Counseling offers emotional support, a means for confronting the issues associated with abuse, and the opportunity for psychological healing. You can find a counselor in your area who specializes in childhood sexual abuse by asking your child's pediatrician or contacting the National Child Abuse Hotline (800–422–4453).

KELLI WATKINS, MD
Gynecology

SEXUALLY TRANSMITTED INFECTIONS (STIs) (e.g., Gonorrhea, Syphilis, Herpes)

Author's Comment: Whatever the specific disease entity might be, it needs to be diagnosed correctly in the doctor's office and treated adequately. Appropriate counseling is definitely advised, and sexual contacts should be sought out and treated if necessary.

1. What are the most common sexually transmitted infections in adolescents?

The most common sexually transmitted infection in the United States is human papilloma virus (HPV). HPV can cause genital warts, cervical dysplasia (precancerous changes on the cervix), and genital cancers including cervical cancer.

Other infections common in adolescents include gonorrhea and chlamydia, which are bacterial infections; *herpes simplex* virus, which is a viral infection; and *Trichomonas vaginalis* which is a protozoan infection. Less common infections in adolescents include hepatitis B, hepatitis C, syphilis, *Pediculosis pubis* ("crabs"), and human immunodeficiency virus (HIV).

2. How are these infections spread?

HPV, herpes, and syphilis can be spread by intercourse, oral sex, or close genital contact. Gonorrhea and chlamydia are more commonly spread by intercourse, but oral sex has resulted in oral and throat infections. Hepatitis B, hepatitis C, and HIV are spread by intercourse (vaginal or anal), needles, and blood transfusions. *Pediculosis pubis* is spread by intercourse, close genital contact, and infected bedding. *Trichomonas* is spread through intercourse.

3. Which infections can be treated or cured?

Bacterial infections (gonorrhea, chlamydia, syphilis) can be treated and cured with antibiotics. *Trichomonas* can also be cured with antibiotics. *Pediculosis pubis* caused by the crab louse is treated and cured with topical medications, removal of nits (eggs), and proper laundering of clothing and bedding. Viral infections such as hepatitis, HPV, and herpes can be cleared by the body. However, sometimes these infections become chronic. Medications can be used to keep symptoms minimal and treat flare-ups but cannot actually cure the infection. HIV attacks the body's immune system. Although medications are available to improve the health and life expectancy of patients with HIV, there is no cure available at this time.

4. Can there be permanent damage from sexually transmitted infections?

Several infections can go on to cause organ damage if not diagnosed and treated. Gonorrhea and chlamydia can lead to scarring of the fallopian tubes, which can result in chronic pelvic pain and infertility. Syphilis can go on to affect the eyes, heart, and nervous system. Chronic hepatitis infections can result in liver failure or liver cancer.

High-risk viral types of human papilloma virus can lead to cervical cancer and other genital cancers. HIV attacks the body's immune system resulting in susceptibility to infections ranging from minor to life threatening.

5. If my child is diagnosed with a sexually transmitted infection, does my child's sexual contact(s) need to be advised?

Sexual partners should be notified when a sexually transmitted infection is diagnosed. Notification will not only allow other potentially affected people to seek evaluation and treatment but also may decrease the likelihood of your child getting reinfected by an untreated partner.

6. What vaccinations are available to prevent sexually transmitted infections?

The hepatitis B vaccine has been part of the routine childhood vaccinations now for many years. A vaccine for the four most common viral types of HPV was approved by the FDA in the spring of 2006. These viral types account for 70 percent of cervical cancer, 50 percent to 60 percent of high-grade dysplasia (precancerous changes on the cervix), and 90 percent of genital warts. The Food and Drug Administration (FDA) has approved the use of this vaccine in girls and young women ages nine to twenty-six years old.

KELLI WATKINS, MD
Gynecology

SHORT STATURE

Definition: Significantly below-average height

Author's Comment: This condition is defined as a height in the lowest 3 percent to 5 percent of the population. Since it is a definition based on statistics, it does not imply a primary health risk but may be a symptom of an underlying health problem. Short stature can have an adverse effect on the child's self-esteem. Supplying information and giving reassurance is especially important to children who experience delayed puberty and have delayed (but not absent) growth.

1. What are the possible causes for this condition?

Many times, short stature is caused by genetics. Short parents tend to have short children. Frequently, short stature is caused by a delay in the timing and duration of growth. In those cases, a child will have his or her pubertal growth spurt later that his or her peer group and grow for a longer period of time; this results in catch-up to normal stature after others have completed their growth.

Occasionally, short stature and slow growth rate can be caused by underlying chronic illness or by malnutrition. Rarely, short stature and slow growth rates are caused by hormonal abnormalities such as hypothyroidism or growth hormone deficiency.

2. What diagnostic tests are needed to define the cause of the short stature?

A careful discussion with your pediatrician and a physical examination will often find genetic or nutritional causes of short stature. Delayed growth, or what is termed "constitutional delay of growth and puberty," can be diagnosed by history, physical examination, and by the use of a bone age X ray of the hand and wrist, which will show a delayed skeletal maturation relative to the chronological age. Additional blood tests may be required to diagnose more subtle chronic illness or hormonal abnormalities such as hypothyroidism or growth hormone deficiency. In addition, measurements over time of the child's height will allow for a determination of the child's pattern of growth. A steady growth rate of 2 inches per year is much less worrisome than a complete cessation of height increase.

3. If the tests indicate a problem, is there anything that can be done to help promote further growth?

Most of the time, short stature is due to genetics or a pattern of delayed growth. These conditions require only close follow-up to monitor the rate of growth and, since they are not a health risk, require no treatment. Any underlying chronic illness related to slow growth rate or short stature should be treated. With adequate treatment, the growth rate may reverse and normal stature may occur.

In the rare cases where a slow growth rate is a symptom of a thyroid hormone or growth hormone deficiency, the missing hormone can be replaced, and the growth pattern can normalize. Growth hormone can also be used in certain genetic conditions, such as Turner syndrome or Prader-Willi syndrome or in chronic renal insufficiency, to promote growth even in the absence of growth hormone deficiency.

Occasionally, growth hormone can be useful to promote growth in children who are at risk of having debilitating short stature as adults, a projected final adult height of less than 59 inches in girls or 63 inches in boys.

4. After all the tests are done, will you be able to give me an estimation of the height that my child will eventually achieve?

This is totally dependent on the cause of the growth problem, if there is one. Many chronic illnesses require treatment that may affect growth rate either positively or negatively, and the course of the illness may be unpredictable. Obviously, in those cases a height prediction using growth charts or other means would be unreliable. In the best circumstances and with consideration of bone age results, height projections are 90 percent accurate within a four-inch range.

5. Do we need to see a pediatric endocrinologist (hormone doctor for children) or any other specialist for an evaluation?

If the child's stature is less than the 3rd to 5th percentile or if the growth rate is less than 2 inches per year in the prepubertal years, a visit to a pediatric endocrinologist is warranted. Any dysmorphic (malformed) features should be evaluated by a geneticist, any malnourished states by a gastroenterologist, and any kidney disease by a nephrologist.

6. What suggestions can you give me so that I personally can help my child deal with this condition?

In the vast majority of cases, short stature is not a symptom of any illness and is just due to genetic or timing issues. Reassurance and emotional support are important, as is careful monitoring of growth rate to ensure that the pattern of growth is normal. An emphasis on healthy lifestyle is also important, and this may include participation in sports. Further encouragement may be necessary if a child chooses to participate in sports that are highly size dependent such as football. Smaller children should be encouraged to work on honing their skills to achieve athletic success rather than the brute force approach to athletic achievement. Alternatively, tennis, golf, soccer, and track are not nearly as size dependent and may allow for excellent exercise and team camaraderie. As with any child, nonathletic interests and talents should also be cultivated to further build self-esteem.

7. How often do you feel it is necessary for you to follow my child's growth in the future?

Your pediatrician will measure and weigh your child at each checkup and plot his or her progress on the growth chart. In most children, this is sufficient to ensure a normal growth pattern. If a potential problem is identified, you may choose to return every six months for a growth follow-up or visit with a pediatric endocrinologist.

ELLEN S. SHER, MD
Endocrinology

SINUSITIS

Definition: Infection of the sinuses.

Author's Comment: Symptoms of sinusitis in childhood may be vague and nonspecific. Frequently there may be only a persistent cough and nasal congestion. The classic headache and green runny nose usually associated with this disease are not always present. Once the condition is diagnosed, however, it is important that a full treatment course be completed as this problem can occur over and over again.

1. What causes sinusitis, and how did my child develop it?

The sinuses are a number of air-filled spaces in the bones of the face that surround and drain into the inside of the nose. At birth these sinuses are very small. They continue to enlarge throughout childhood and are not fully developed until late adolescence. There are four paired sets of sinuses. The maxillary sinuses are large spaces located behind the cheek between the upper teeth and the eyes. The ethmoid sinuses are a series of small cavities between the eyes. The frontal sinuses are in the forehead. The sphenoid sinuses are deep inside the head, at the back of the nose.

Sinusitis is inflammation, swelling, and/or infection of the sinuses. Sinusitis can be acute, chronic, or recurrent acute.

- Acute sinusitis most commonly includes "cold-like symptoms" (congested nose, runny nose, postnasal drip, bad breath, or cough) that persist without improvement beyond ten days. The cold-like symptoms typically get worse seven to ten days after they start in children with acute sinusitis. A fever and/or green runny nasal discharge are not always present in children with acute sinusitis.

- Chronic sinusitis is a low-grade infection lasting more than three months and involving symptoms such as nasal obstruction, congestion, runny nose, postnasal drip, cough, bad breath, and/or headache. In chronic sinusitis the lining of the sinuses thickens, and obstructing tissue known as polyps may develop.

- Recurrent acute sinusitis is four or more episodes of acute sinusitis per year, each lasting at least ten days, with healthy intervals between episodes.

Children average between six and eight upper respiratory infections ("colds") per year, 5 percent to 10 percent of which are complicated by acute sinusitis.

2. What diagnostic tests need to better define the condition?

The diagnosis of acute sinusitis is not always easy to make, since the common symptoms in children—nasal obstruction, runny nose and cough—are very much the same as those of a simple cold. Children rarely have the facial pain that adults will get with acute sinusitis. X rays are not usually helpful, since clouding of the sinuses on plain X rays or even a CAT scan is a common finding in children with colds. Very young children may have abnormal sinus X rays even if they have no infection at all. X rays or CAT scans should be reserved for situations in which the patient does not recover or worsens during the course of antibiotic therapy. Cultures of the nose can also be misleading, since they do not reflect the actual contents of the sinuses. Therefore, children with cold symptoms lasting more than ten days can simply be assumed to have sinusitis and treated. The diagnosis may be made earlier if facial pain is present, or if there is a complication of sinusitis (such as spread of infection to the eye).

Children with chronic symptoms of sinusitis (lasting more than a few months) are usually treated with a variety of medications as outlined below. If medical management is unsuccessful in relieving symptoms, a CAT scan may be useful if surgery is being considered. This scan will accurately depict the anatomy and any inflammation in the sinus cavities.

3. How is it treated?

The following are treatment options:

Acute sinusitis is treated with antibiotics, usually for a two- to three-week course. A short course of nasal decongestant spray (no more than three days) may be helpful to open the sinus drainage pathways and allow the infection to clear more rapidly.

Chronic sinusitis can be helped by nasal steroid sprays, which reduce inflammation and swelling. These sprays are fairly safe and are not absorbed in significant amounts. Therefore, they do not have the same side effects as steroids taken by mouth and can be used for prolonged periods of time. Antibiotics are also given to these patients to treat the bacteria that may be contributing to congestion, inflammation, and polyp formation.

If there is an allergic component to the nasal disease, specific allergy treatment (such as antihistamines) may be useful. However, if allergy is not present, the use of antihistamines is not recommended. Many of these drugs have drying effects on the lining of the nose, which interferes with the body's ability to keep the nose clean and to eliminate bacteria and other debris. Also, some of the agents approved for use in young children may have undesirable behavioral side effects.

One very effective and safe treatment for both acute and chronic sinusitis is to keep nasal passages moist through the use of humidification and nasal irrigation. Keeping the lining of the nose moist is important to the body's own natural defenses. Moisture also keeps the nasal secretions from drying out and blocking the natural sinus drainage pathways. Room humidifiers are helpful, but care must be taken to keep them clean, or they can grow colonies of bacteria and/or fungus. Nasal saline spray should be used frequently as well.

Sinus surgery is rarely recommended for young children. The goal of sinus surgery is to remove bone and other tissue that are blocking the natural sinus drainage pathways, allowing the sinuses to return to health. Nasal disease in young children is often more complicated than simple blockage of the sinus "bottleneck" and may be the result of a number of factors such as an immature immune system, frequent exposure to colds and viruses, poor nasal hygiene, and enlarged adenoids. Surgery may be appropriate for a few selected children who have significant symptoms that cannot be controlled by medical management.

4. Are there any potential side effects from the treatment?

Any therapy has potential side effects. Treatment with antibiotics has the potential for the development of diarrhea, nausea, vomiting, rash, or allergic reaction. Treatment with antihistamines or steroid nose sprays may lead to nasal dryness and even nose bleeds. The risk of surgeries should be discussed with your surgeon.

5. Can the disorder be possibly allergy related, and, if so, what can be done about it?

Yes. An allergy is a condition in which the body responds to some foreign substance such as dust, pollen, fungus, mold, or certain medications. The substance causing the allergic reaction is called an allergen. The reaction can be mild (for example, a rash) or severe and life threatening. In nasal allergy, the nose responds to an inhaled allergen by increasing the normal output of mucous and by swelling shut internally. This results in a sensation of nasal obstruction and nasal drainage, similar to sinusitis. The symptoms of nasal allergies are different from sinusitis in that they may start suddenly after exposure to the allergen, the drainage is usually thin and clear, and there is generally no facial pain. Furthermore, allergic children often have other symptoms such as watery eyes, itching, rashes, and hives.

Allergies are treated with antihistamines, steroid nasal sprays, and other prescribed medications. Allergy testing can identify the specific allergen (what your child is allergic to). Allergy shots (immunotherapy) are the only potential cure for allergies and are specifically directed to the findings of your child's allergy testing.

6. Will an X ray be needed at the end of the treatment to make sure the sinus infection is completely gone?

Typically no; the diagnosis of acute sinusitis should be based on the child's history and physical findings. Likewise, the resolution of acute sinusitis should be based on clinical criteria. In situations where a child has chronic sinusitis or recurrent acute sinusitis, a CAT scan may be needed after medical therapy to assess resolution of the disease.

7. What can be done to prevent this condition from recurring in the future?

This depends on the cause of the sinus infection. In children with recurrent upper respiratory viral infections that lead to bacterial sinusitis, the practice of good sanitary habits is advisable. Avoidance of close physical contact and not sharing of napkins, towels, and utensils with infected children will decrease their risk of illness. Frequent hand washing makes good sense.

In individuals that have known environmental allergies, good medical control of the allergies combined with avoidance (when possible) of the allergen can decrease the recurrence of sinusitis.

Surgically removing adenoids to relieve obstruction of the normal drainage pathways and remove a source of bacterial contamination of the nose may decrease the recurrence of sinusitis in select children. The use of sinus surgery to open the normal drainage pathways of the sinuses or relieve anatomic obstruction can also be effective in preventing recurrence.

8. Do we need to see a specialist for this type of disorder?

The specialists that are typically involved with the care of sinusitis are otolaryngologists (ear, nose, and throat doctors) and/or allergists.

Timing of referral to a specialist will be determined by your primary care physician based on your child's individual history and symptoms. Children that do not get better with treatment or have chronic sinus infections or have significant, recurrent, acute sinus infections should be seen by a specialist. Children with complete nasal obstruction that does not respond to medical therapy should also be seen by a specialist. Children with any complication from sinusitis should be evaluated by a specialist as soon as possible.

9. When do you wish to see my child again for a follow-up?

Children are typically seen again after four weeks to assess response to medical therapy.

PAUL W. BAUER, MD
Otolaryngology

SKIN INFECTION
(Impetigo and Cellulitis)

Definition: **Superficial infection of the skin.**

Author's Comment: This condition is very common in childhood. Children are constantly getting scrapes and insect bites that can then become infected. The high frequency of occurrence emphasizes the need for good hand-washing techniques to be encouraged in all children.

1. What causes this condition, and how did my child contract it?

There are two main forms of skin infection: impetigo and cellulitis. Impetigo is a bacterial infection of the top layer of the skin, usually caused by strep and/or staph bacteria. If there is not a great deal of redness of the surrounding skin, it can often be treated with antibiotic creams applied topically. Cellulitis is an infection of the deeper layers of the skin and is potentially more serious. It is manifested by a spreading redness of the skin.

Children usually get impetigo from a scratch or abrasion that gets infected with a bacteria that happens to be on the skin. Cellulitis can occur as a result of spread of impetigo, or it can be a result of a deeper infection that spreads toward the skin.

2. Is it contagious, and, if so, what can I do to prevent its spread?

The skin infection itself is not contagious, but the bacteria that cause it can be spread to someone else, especially if it is a staph or strep bacteria. In another person, however, it may cause no infection, or possibly an infection at a different site, if at all.

3. What is the treatment for this condition?

For mild impetigo, treatment of the involved area with an antibiotic cream will often be effective, but, for more severe forms of impetigo or for cellulitis, oral or injection antibiotics are usually used.

4. Are there any side effects from the medicines used for the treatment that I should be aware of?

For topical antibiotic creams, there are few side effects unless a person is allergic to the cream. For oral or injectable antibiotics, there are more possible side effects such as diarrhea, vomiting, allergic reactions, and the possibility of development of resistance to antibiotics for the bacteria causing infection and for other bacteria on the child's body.

5. Is this the type of disorder that can recur?

Yes. There is practically no immunity that a person develops to this type of infection. After a bout of impetigo, a person can contract it again after another scratch or abrasion, if certain bacteria are present on the skin.

6. What advice should be given to people who have been in contact with my child?

Since the bacteria that cause impetigo can cause other types of infections, people who have been in contact with your child should watch for signs of infection, but there are no special things that are necessary unless your child has an infection with an unusual strain of bacteria. Your doctor can tell you if the bacteria causing your child's infection is particularly contagious or not; most are not.

7. Are there potential complications from this disorder?

The infection can occasionally spread from the skin to other parts of the body. The most serious of these are infections that spread to the bloodstream, where the infection can potentially go anywhere in the body. Fortunately, this is rare with impetigo, but it happens more often with cellulitis. Rarely, skin infection can lead to a kidney complication called glomerulonephritis, which is the result of an immune response to certain strains of strep infection.

8. When should I see improvement in my child?

There should be improvement within one to two days. If you see no improvement at all, or worsening, contact your child's doctor again.

9. Do you need to see my child again for this condition?

If the condition is not improving within a few days, or if your child gets sicker, you should contact your doctor.

GREGORY R. ISTRE, MD
Infectious Diseases

SLEEP DISORDERS
(e.g., Night Terrors, Nightmares, Difficulty Getting to Sleep, Sleepwalking)

Definition: Conditions that disrupt or interfere with the sleep process.

Author's Comment: These maddening conditions can lead to many sleepless nights on the part of the child and parents. Consult your doctor regarding any specific medication or behavioral modification that can possibly alter the course of these conditions.

1. What causes these sleep disorders?

Some events such as night terrors and sleepwalking can run in families. These disorders, in particular, occur during the deepest stages of sleep, meaning that the child does not remember the event in the morning. Although there are no direct negative effects to the child from these occurrences, safety measures are imperative. Protecting your child from stairways or from leaving the home is essential.

Sleepwalking or night terror events frequently occur on nights that the child is "overtired" or abnormally stressed. Nightmares and difficulty getting to sleep occur occasionally in normal children but should be investigated with your pediatrician if they occur nightly for more than two weeks.

2. What dangers are posed by this condition?

Night terrors and sleepwalking can include nonsensical speaking and walking around the house. Although not indicative of deeper illness, injuries can occur due to clumsy, noncoordinated movements. Staircases should be gated off, pool gates locked, and doors leading to the outdoors should be bolted out of reach.

3. What tests need to be done to better define this condition?

After speaking with your pediatrician, he or she may refer you to a pediatric sleep medicine specialist. An overnight test called a polysomnogram may be considered. This test occurs in a specialized sleep laboratory and monitors such things as your child's heart rate, breathing rate and pattern, oxygenation level, body movements, and brain waves. Analysis of this information may help discern the "trigger" for nighttime conditions such as sleepwalking and can help confirm the presence or absence of normal nighttime respirations.

4. Is there any treatment?

If abnormal nocturnal breathing is identified, the most common treatment is surgical removal of the adenoids and tonsils. This "cures" sleep-disordered breathing in around 80 percent of the cases. If breathing is normal but sleep disruption still occurs, oral medication or behavioral therapies may be prescribed.

5. Are there any potential side effects that can occur from the treatment?

Surgical removal of the adenoids and tonsils carries the typical risks for surgery. Any medication use will have its own set of side effects that should be discussed by your physician.

6. Do you suggest any adjustments in my family's lifestyle that should take place?

Beyond having a set bedtime and set waketime for your child, other helpful sleep hints include the limiting of caffeinated beverages, limiting active computer or video game usage just prior to bedtime, and helping your child to be self-calming. Many children that have difficulty sleeping have trouble "quieting their minds" to allow sleep. This is a learned skill and can be discussed as a family. Children who sleepwalk or have night terrors should be made safe and not ridiculed. Since the children do not remember the event and cannot control it, discussion in a negative tone can cause damage to a child's self-esteem.

7. Will my child outgrow this condition and, if so, when?

Most children outgrow night terrors and sleepwalking by the time they enter puberty.

8. Do we need to consult a specialist, such as a psychologist or sleep disorder clinic?

If your pediatrician feels that your child's nighttime events are out of the range of normal (such as increased frequency or intensity), or if the events are changing for the worse, consultation with a pediatric sleep medicine physician should occur to rule out physical abnormalities. You then may be referred to a psychologist if the physician feels that behavioral therapy may benefit your child. In cases of insomnia, eight to twelve visits with a therapist can "teach" your child to be a better sleeper. Sometimes normal bedtime fears can escalate into insomnia or insistence on sleeping with the parents. These issues can also be worked on with a therapist who specializes in pediatric bedtime issues.

9. When do you wish to see my child again regarding this disorder?

Pediatricians should be kept informed of the therapies or medication trials used to help with sleep disorders. Follow-up may occur with the psychologist, sleep specialist, or simply your pediatrician. A specific plan will be worked out among those providers.

HILARY PEARSON, MD
Sleep Medicine

SMALL HEAD
(Microcephaly)

Author's Comment: Pediatricians measure the head circumference at every routine visit during the child's infancy to pick up conditions such as this. It is worrisome when a child's head is not growing adequately. Your child's doctor will advise you on which diagnostic tests are necessary and what to do next.

1. What caused this condition?

Microcephaly is defined as the head size being less than two standard deviations below the average. This is normal for approximately 5 percent of children. Also this can be a sign of a problem with brain growth.

If there is abnormal brain growth it can be caused by infections of the baby before birth, genetic defects, or toxic exposure (such as alcohol or radiation). In addition, bone problems can cause microcephaly, when the spaces between the bones of the skull close prematurely (craniosynostosis).

2. How will this condition affect my child's learning and intellectual function?

If the brain's growth is abnormal children can have cognitive defects, attention difficulties, or movement problems (cerebral palsy). Thirty percent may have epilepsy.

3. What diagnostic tests are needed to further establish the cause and define the condition?

Depending on the history and physical examination, tests such as an MRI of the brain, an EEG (electroencephalogram), as well as genetic and metabolic testing may be useful.

4. What is the proposed treatment for this condition, and how successful is it?

If a specific metabolic defect is found there may be a specific treatment. Otherwise, treatment is based on what other problems the child has, typically physical therapy for cerebral palsy or medications for epilepsy.

5. What specialist should we consult and when?

When the problem becomes apparent, specialists that could help include pediatric neurologists, geneticists, and physical medicine and rehabilitation specialists, as well as developmental pediatricians.

6. Could this condition affect future children we might have?

If the cause of the microcephaly is found to be genetic in nature this could recur in other children.

7. When do you wish to see my child again regarding this condition?

Follow-up with the pediatrician depends on what other problems the child has and how severe these problems are.

DAVID B. OWEN, MD
Neurology

SPITTING UP
(Gastroesophageal Reflux—GER)

Definition: An effortless backflow of stomach
               contents into the mouth due to an incom-
               petent, malfunctioning valve that sepa-
               rates the stomach from the esophagus
               (swallowing tube).

Author's Comment: This is one of the most common problems pediatricians deal with during the child's first year of life. Many medicines
and formula changes might be tried at times with only variable
success. The encouraging fact is that 80 percent of children outgrow
this condition by the time they are eighteen months of age.

1. What causes this condition?
The most common cause of GER in infancy and young childhood is
the temporary relaxation of the lower esophageal sphincter (LES) and
associated abnormal movement of the esophagus. The LES is the
connection from the esophagus to the stomach. It is not a muscle flap
but simply a smooth muscle that is contracted (closed) in the resting
state. There are anatomical differences in length and position from

infants to adults that may account for the increased number of reflux episodes that tend to occur in children under twelve years of age.

There can be other anatomical causes for reflux, such as abnormal movement of the esophagus and congenital defects. GER is increased in preterm infants, patients with chronic lung disease (bronchopulmonary disease [BPD] or cystic fibrosis [CF]), and neurologically impaired patients with abnormal muscle tone.

2. What symptoms and complications can occur because of it?

The most common symptom of GER is regurgitation. This means the passage of stomach contents into the throat and mouth. Vomiting is defined as the expulsion of the stomach contents from the mouth. Once there is development of symptoms, GER becomes gastroesophageal reflux disease (GERD).

In other words, when it comes to spitting up, there are happy spitters and then there are others who may have symptoms such as heartburn, feeding difficulties such as refusal to eat, taking only small amounts or crying during feeding, poor weight gain, and pulmonary symptoms such as wheezing, apnea, and/or pneumonia. Significant complications from GERD consist of inflammation of the esophagus, narrowing of the esophagus, vomiting blood, failure to thrive (not gaining weight appropriately), and other issues such as recurrent sinusitis, vocal cord nodules, and Barrett's esophagus (a precancerous lesion).

3. How is this condition treated and for how long?

The treatment of GER or GERD is based upon the severity of the symptoms. For the happy spitter it is simply reassurance. Due to the anatomical differences in children versus adults, all infants reflux to some degree. It is well documented that reflux worsens between the ages of four to six months. By twelve to fifteen months of age greater than 95 percent of infants have complete resolution of their symptoms. For these children, offering small, frequent feedings and elevating the head of the bed by a 30-degree angle is warranted.

If the infant/child has irritability, feeding difficulties or poor weight gain more aggressive treatment in warranted. A trial of H2 blockers (ranitidine, famotidine) or a proton pump inhibitor (PPI), such as lansoprazole or omeprazole, is initiated. If there is poor response to treatment, other options include the use of a prokinetic agent (gastrointestinal or esophageal muscle stimulant) such as metoclopramide or bethanecol. The medication doses are based upon the weight of the child and are adjusted rather frequently due to the rapid weight gain in the first fifteen months of life. The medication is used until the child shows improvement and/or resolution of the symptoms. Usually, one lets the child "outgrow" the medication dosage and watches for any new signs or symptoms to develop.

4. How effective is the treatment, and, if medicines are used, what are the potential side effects that can occur?

Lifestyle changes are effective treatment in approximately 50 percent of children. The effectiveness of H2 blockers for the healing of esophagitis (inflammation, irritation to the esophagus) is approximately 60 percent but with the use of PPIs it is greater than 85 percent.

Side effects from H2 blockers include headache, abdominal pain, and constipation. The most common side effects from the use of PPIs are headache, rash, abdominal pain, and constipation. These occur in less than 6 percent of the people. This data is similar to placebo (sugar pill). There have been no reported long-term side effects with the use of PPIs.

Side effects from the use of prokinetic agents such as metoclopramide and bethanecol are more significant, and the benefit must outweigh the risk. Metoclopramide works by increasing the resting LES pressure and increasing the rate of stomach emptying. Side effects occur in 11 percent to 35 percent of people and range from drowsiness and restlessness to the most significant reaction called acute dystonic reaction. This can include neck rigidity, shaking, and seizure-like activity. It is treated with withdrawal of the medication and/or diphenhydramine. Bethanecol increases the LES pressure. It has similar but less severe side effects than metoclopramide.

5. How do I guard against my child choking or aspirating when lying on the back?

Infants with GER should receive small, frequent feedings, reducing the amount of formula in the stomach that is available to reflux. It is important that infants are kept upright at a 30-degree angle for thirty to forty-five minutes after meals and that they are burped well. When laying the infant on the back, attempts should be made to turn the head to one side (alternating sides) and limit bedding near the head and face region.

If there is choking occurring despite these measures, other issues must be considered. This would include swallowing abnormalities with aspiration. For this to be evaluated, a modified barium swallow (a type of X ray study) would be performed. This can be ordered by your primary care physician or pediatric gastroenterologist.

6. What are the chances that my child will outgrow this disorder with or without treatment?

In most cases, infants with GER or GERD will outgrow the condition by fifteen to eighteen months of age. There are some children who will continue to exhibit ongoing issues of reflux such as heartburn, regurgitation, and pain in the upper abdominal region. These particular patients have periods of their symptoms waxing and waning but never resolving. There is typically a family history of reflux. They require long term treatment with lifestyle changes and/or medications. They should be evaluated and followed by a pediatric gastroenterologist.

7. Do we need to be referred to a doctor who specializes in this condition?

Referrals should be made to a pediatric gastroenterologist when there are complications from the GER. This includes feeding difficulties, vomiting blood, poor weight gain, significant irritability, and/or poor response to treatment. It is important to keep your primary care physician informed of any formula changes, lifestyle changes, or medications.

8. What symptoms or signs would warrant my calling you back?

If there are any changes that have taken place since the last visit to the office, the physician should be notified. These can include increased regurgitation, irritability, change in feeding habits, change in sleep habits, feeding difficulties such as gagging or choking, vomiting blood, and/or increased pulmonary symptoms (cough, congestion, asthma).

9. When do you wish to see my child again regarding this condition?

The child should be evaluated on a two to six month basis. Young infants with significant GERD may need to be seen every few weeks. It is important that is the first year of life they are seen every two to six months to see how they are progressing with feedings, severity of symptoms, and their growth pattern. The physician will be able to guide you through the different stages of feeding and growth. There are times that infants require feeding therapy with an occupational therapist due to the development of feeding problems from significant reflux.

ANNETTE WHITNEY, MD
Gastroenterology

SPRAIN OF EXTREMITY (e.g., Toe, Ankle, Knee, Finger, Wrist, Elbow)

Definition: The straining of a joint with partial rupture or other injury of its attachment.

Author's Comment: This condition occurs often in childhood and adolescence as children are frequently putting their bodies at risk in various forms of play or exercise. Consult your child's doctor when you suspect a sprain has occurred. Most of these conditions get better with rest alone, but some of the severe ones need orthopedic follow-up.

1. What is a sprain?

A sprain is when the tissues supporting a joint (ligaments or tendons) become stretched and injured. This can occur from the tendons being pulled or ligaments being stretched or completely torn. The pain and swelling that result is around a joint.

Sometimes a sprain can be confused with a fracture because it occurs in the bony area. If not diagnosed and treated properly, a sprain can cause long-term problems. It is important to distinguish a sprain from a fracture. The age of the child and the manner in which the limb was injured are important in determining a sprain or fracture.

Children under the age of eight years very rarely truly sprain a joint and are much more likely to actually break something.

2. What is the treatment for this condition?

The treatment for a sprain involves resting of the involved area and typically splinting. Splinting is a means to hold the area still, and this allows the ligaments or tendons that have been stretched or possibly partially torn to heal at the proper length. If a tendon or ligament stretched heals in a stretched-out position, it will never return to its original length.

A sprain takes typically six weeks to heal. Unfortunately, a sprain is painful for the first seven to ten days. The pain, thereafter, typically goes away, and the natural tendency at this point is to stop treating the sprain because the pain has resolved. However, it is important to continue to treat the sprain for at least four to six weeks. Even if the pain is resolved, the tendons or ligaments are still healing.

The treatment includes splinting either with a splint or cast, custom applied or purchased over the counter. Once the injury has healed, the joint often feels stiff. The age of the child, the injury location, the number of sprains, and the desire to return to sporting activities will determine if physical therapy is needed.

3. Are X ray studies needed to make sure there is no fracture?

In growing children, the ligaments that support the joint attach to the bones at the ends of the bones. This is very close to the area where the growth plates are located. X rays are important in young children to help distinguish a sprain from a growth plate fracture. A more important aspect is the careful physical examination. If this joint is tender over the joint area itself and not over the bony area, this fits with the diagnosis of a sprain. If there is tenderness on the bony ends or with pushing directly on the bone itself, the likelihood of a fracture is high. X rays are important to see if there is a break that is visible on the X ray.

If an X ray is performed and no break is visualized, this does not mean that a fracture does not exist. In growing children, fractures of the growth plate, which is a visible gap on the X ray, are often misdiagnosed as sprains. Growth plate fractures are hard to diagnose if the bone has not shifted. It is not always accurate to diagnose a sprain just simply with a physical examination.

4. How long will the discomfort last?

Typically with a sprain, most of the discomfort is within the first seven to ten days. At two weeks from date of injury, most of the pain should be resolved. If pain lasts longer than two weeks, it is important to be evaluated.

Although the discomfort will improve, the sprain itself actually takes four to six weeks to completely heal. Healing is not just the absence of pain.

5. What is the timetable for resuming activities that involve the injured part of the body?

Children should wait four to six weeks from the date of the injury before resuming normal activities. This is the length of time that is needed to allow the soft tissues to appropriately heal.

6. Is there a possibility that there will be any permanent disability?

If the sprain is diagnosed early and if the area is rested properly so that the stretched ligaments and joint can heal in its normal position and length, there should be no permanent disability. However, if the sprain is not treated appropriately and allowed to heal stretched out, if the individual returns to activities too soon, and the joint is reinjured soon after being injured initially, this can cause the joint to become permanent loosened, in which case this could become a permanent disability. If not a disability, this could become a permanent loosening of the joint, which would then lead to a high chance of having recurring injuries in the future.

7. Do you think it is necessary to consult an orthopedist?

Your pediatrician is the person best trained to see initially with this problem. With his or her knowledge of you, your child, and medicine, he or she can best decide when a referral is needed.

Having said this, an orthopedist can be quite helpful in the treatment of severe sprains. If a sprain is not allowed to heal properly, it can cause long-term problems. Sprains sometimes really are fractures that are misdiagnosed, especially in the pediatric population. It is important to follow up with your pediatrician or an orthopedist about one to two weeks following the initial injury to ensure that symptoms are improving with time. Obviously, if there is an injury that has been diagnosed as a sprain and is not usable at all, it is important to seek an orthopedist much sooner.

8. When should I bring my child back for a follow-up exam?

Sprains typically heal in six weeks. It is important that they are properly diagnosed. Your child should be seen soon after the injury and then seven to ten days later. If the pediatrician or primary care physician refers you to see an orthopedist, this visit should take place seven to ten days following the injury, or sooner if there is a lot of swelling, pain, or suspicion of a fracture. Discussion of physical therapy is appropriate seven to ten days following the injury. In most cases, physical therapy will not begin until after six weeks. Early physical therapy, however, can help diminish swelling and improve comfort depending on the age of the child and the joint involved.

Six weeks from injury, a follow-up examination should be made to ensure there is no pain, swelling, tenderness, or instability of the joint. At six weeks from date of injury if there is no pain, swelling, tenderness, or instability of the joint, the sprain has healed, and the child can resume normal activities. If the child is a highly competitive athlete, such as a gymnast, it would be advantageous to consider physical therapy, taping, or bracing prior to resuming a high-stress sport. This decision can best be made in conjunction with the orthopedist and the child six weeks following the injury.

W. BARRY HUMENIUK, MD
Orthopedics

STYE

Definition: An inflammation of an eyelid gland.

Author's Comment: This condition usually clears up with localized treatment. Realize, though, that the condition can progress and involve the entire eyelid, warranting more generalized treatment.

1. What causes this condition to occur, and how did my child contract it?

A style results from an infection of an eyelid gland. It is typically not contagious.

2. What complications can occur because of it?

If the infection progresses, a more severe infection involving swelling and redness of the eye and eyelids may occur.

3. How is it treated, and are antibiotics indicated?

Antibiotics are frequently used to treat a stye. Most frequently this involves antibiotic ointment or drops. Oral antibiotics may also be used. Warm compresses may also be helpful.

4. What are the potential side effects of the treatment?

Side effects of treatment may occur due to an allergic reaction to the medicine, or there may be irritation of the eye or eyelid caused by the medicine.

5. Are any isolation precautions necessary because of this condition?

Isolation precautions are typically not necessary.

6. How long does it take for this condition to resolve?

Most styes will resolve within one week with treatment.

7. What signs would warrant my getting back in touch with you?

Progression of swelling, fever, or severe pain warrant further consultation with your doctor.

8. When do you wish to see my child again for this condition?

If symptoms progress after two or three days of treatment, you should contact your doctor. If the swelling and redness resolve with treatment, it is not necessary to consult with your doctor.

DAVID STAGER, JR, MD
Ophthalmology

TEAR DUCT OBSTRUCTION
(Nasolacrimal Obstruction)

Definition: A blocked or partially blocked duct in the tear apparatus.

Author's Comment: This condition causes recurrent discharge from the eye during the first months of life. It is a common occurrence during infancy. Most of the time the condition responds to a conservative treatment plan prescribed by your child's doctor. If not, the child may need to see an ophthalmologist (eye specialist) for further intervention.

1. What causes this condition, and how did my child develop it?

Tear duct (nasolacrimal) obstruction is commonly a congenital condition that occurs in 5 percent to 6 percent of newborn infants. It is usually the result of a blockage or incomplete opening at the lower end of the tear duct. More rarely, it may occur because of the incomplete development of the nasolacrimal system.

2. What are the complications that might occur as a result of it?

Typically, affected infants will have an overflow of tears, wet-looking eyes, a pus-like discharge, or lower eyelid irritation. Unlike conjunctivitis ("pink eye") the eyes are usually not red. Chronic or recurring eye infections may occur as a result of this condition.

3. Can the vision be affected in any way?

Vision is not at risk as a result of this condition. However, if the tear sac becomes infected and is untreated, a more serious infection may occur that could affect vision.

4. What is the treatment?

A high percentage of blocked tear ducts will open with local massage of the nasolacrimal sac. Antibiotic drops or ointment can be used to treat the discharge. If the symptoms have not improved by age six months to one year, infants can undergo a simple office procedure, probing of the nasolacrimal duct. Excessive tearing and discharge may indicate the need for earlier probing.

5. What are the chances for success as a result of the treatment?

Within the first year of life, 85 percent to 90 percent of tear duct obstructions may clear with conservative management (massage, topical antibiotics). Nasolacrimal probings, if necessary, have the highest success rate when performed within the first year of life.

6. What symptoms would warrant my contacting you again regarding this condition?

Your doctor should be contacted if your child has a continued over-flow of tears, mucous discharge, lid irritation, or chronic conjunctivitis (red eye).

7. When do you wish to see my child again for reevaluation of this disorder?

By age six to twelve months, if conservative management has not opened the tear duct, additional treatments such as a tear duct probing should be considered.

JOEL LEFFLER, MD
Ophthalmology

THRUSH

Definition: A fungal disease of infants characterized by whitish patches in the mouth and on the tongue.

Author's Comment: This condition often looks worse than it actually is. Sometimes more than one round of medicine is needed to make it go away. Also, if you are a nursing mom, be careful! You might contract the infection on your breast.

1. What is the cause of this condition, and how did my child contract it?

Thrush is a common condition that occurs mostly in healthy infants. It is caused by a yeast-type fungal infection of the mucous membranes that line the mouth. The fungus is called *Candida*. It produces an infection of this area of the mouth and results in white patches on the lining of the mouth and the tongue. It may cause some discomfort, especially when feeding.

Many healthy infants get this infection for no apparent reason; some contract it after taking antibiotics. Thrush is the result of overgrowth of the fungus, which are present in almost everyone's mouth but which are usually kept in check by the normal bacteria that are present the mouth. Antibiotics can decrease the number of bacteria, resulting in overgrowth of the fungus in some cases, similar to the way that some women can get yeast infections of the vagina after taking antibiotics. Rarely, if the condition is severe or prolonged, it may represent an underlying immune problem in the child, but the vast majority of infants who get thrush are otherwise healthy.

2. Is it contagious, and, if so, how is it spread?

The infection itself is not contagious, but the yeast that causes it can be spread to someone else, although it usually does not cause infection in older children or adults. Occasionally, a breastfeeding mother may get a mild infection similar to thrush on her breast. Thorough cleaning can help prevent this from happening.

3. Does it cause any discomfort during feeding?

Thrush may cause some discomfort for the infant during feedings and often is the first sign that the infant has thrush.

4. Is there any problem with my child's immune system that may have led to the development of this condition?

Most of the time, thrush occurs in otherwise healthy infants. Only in severe cases, or cases that are protracted or recurrent, is there a greater chance of an immune problem.

5. What is the treatment for this disorder?

For mild thrush, sometimes no treatment is necessary. For more involved cases, your doctor may prescribe a mycostatin solution to apply to the lining of the mouth and tongue or an oral medication to take for a brief time.

6. Are there side effects from the medicines used for the treatment that I should be aware of?

For topical solutions, there are few side effects unless a person is allergic to it. For oral antifungals, possible side effects include diarrhea, vomiting, allergic reactions, and the development of resistance to the antifungal.

7. How long does it take for the condition to improve with treatment?

Usually the initial response is within a day or two, with complete clearing within two weeks.

8. Can the condition spread to any other parts of the body?

Any area of the body that is moist and covered (such as the diaper area, the armpits, etc.) can develop a similar yeast infection, especially after the child has taken antibiotics.

9. If I am nursing my baby, is there any particular prescription to apply to my breasts to prevent my contracting this disorder?

There are several available, but they are usually not needed because most women do not develop infection on the breast, especially if care is taken to clean the breast well after feeding and the area is kept dry.

10. What symptoms or signs would warrant my calling you back and when?

If the white patches do not go away after a few days of treatment, or if they worsen substantially or recur soon after treatment, or if your infant does not feed well, then you should call your pediatrician for advice.

11. Do you wish to recheck my child for this condition?

If the condition is not improving within a few days, or if your child gets sicker, or if the thrush recurs, please call your pediatrician.

GREGORY R. ISTRE, MD
Infectious Diseases

TIC DISORDERS

Definition: Involuntary movements of certain muscle groups of the body.

Author's Comment: These sudden muscle jerks or twitches that characterize tics can be socially disconcerting for the patient and onlookers.

1. What are tics?

Tics are somewhat involuntary, quick, repetitive movements, vocalizations, or sensations. Usually they are one or a few stereotypic movements (the same thing over and over). These can change over the course of time. These movements can be suppressed but only temporarily and with effort. Tics can be simple or complex, most tics are temporary and insignificant. Less often they are long-standing major problems to a patient.

2. What causes tics?

The exact reasons for tics are still unknown. There does seem to be an imbalance or over sensitivity to certain neurotransmitters in the brain. Genetics is a strong factor but other factors can play a role as well, such as infections. Tics are not seizures.

3. Can a child be taught not to do the tic?
No. Even though it can be temporarily suppressed people should not punish someone for having a tic, this possibly would make the tic even worse. Relaxation training is sometimes helpful. Teachers and coaches should be told about tics so that the child is not punished or the tics misinterpreted.

4. What treatments are available?
Often no treatment is needed. If the tics are causing problems for the child, medications such as alpha blockers or dopamine blockers can be tried. The main side effect of these medicines is sedation, which is usually temporary. Constipation can also be a side effect. Dopamine blockers can cause weight gain.

Again, some people benefit from relaxation training. If there are other problems, such as obsessive-compulsive disorder, attention deficit hyperactivity disorder (ADHD), depression, sleep disturbance, anxiety, or aggressive disorder, medication may be helpful.

5. What is Tourette's syndrome?
Tics vary quite a bit as far as severity and long term prognosis. Most cases of tics are simple tics and are temporary (just a year or so). These are not enough of a problem for the child to be on medication. Five to 15 percent of elementary school children, especially boys, have transient tics. Chronic tics are tics that last greater than a year and are severe enough to cause problems.

Tourette's syndrome is a chronic neuropsychiatric disorder that includes chronic severe motor and vocal tics. Often these are accompanied by many of the other problems listed in question #4. Tourette's syndrome accounts for less than 10 percent of patients with motor tics. Tourette's syndrome and chronic motor tics wax and wane in severity with time. Sometimes this condition gets better on its own.

6. What doctors should be involved in the care of tic patients?

Often the pediatrician or family doctor can diagnose temporary, simple motor tics. If the tics are causing significant problems for the child, a pediatric neurologist or child psychiatrist or psychologist are needed. Some testing may be needed if the child's case is not clear cut.

7. What follow-up is needed?

Follow-up is dependent on the condition of the patient. If a patient is placed on medication such as the alpha blockers or dopamine blockers, more frequent follow-up would be required.

DAVID B. OWEN, MD
Neurology

TONSILLITIS

Definition: **Inflammation of the tonsils.**

Author's Comment: When your child complains of a sore throat, possibly accompanied by fever, you need to take the child to the doctor to have the throat cultured so as to rule out the possibility of strep. If the child has strep, you will receive medicine to treat the condition. This is the way it has been done for decades.

1. What causes this condition?

A sore throat (pharyngitis) can be caused by a number of problems, but it is usually the result of a virus infecting the upper respiratory tract (the mouth, nose, and throat). The vast majority of cases of sore throat are related to viral infections. Less commonly, sore throats can be caused by a bacterial infection. Strep throat is the most common bacteria that can cause tonsillitis. Strep is an infection by one particular type of bacteria. Many other types of bacteria can cause throat infections. Most doctors will try to specifically diagnose the strep bacteria with a throat swab, because in rare cases, these infections can result in damage to the heart or kidneys.

When tonsils are infected with bacteria, they will usually get large, turn somewhat red, and may have some yellowish-white debris on the surface. Appearances can be misleading, as there are some viruses that can make the tonsils look like this (as in mononucleosis—"mono"). The strep bacteria can be present in a normal-looking throat. The only way to be sure is to do a throat culture (throat swab).

2. Is it contagious, and how did my child contract it?

Most throat infections are contagious. Viral throat infections are spread by close contact because the viruses are present in nose secretions (snot) and saliva. The use of objects such as utensils, cups, or a child's teething item where the secretions or saliva are present in heavy concentrations may also cause spread. Bacterial throat infections with strep are also contracted by close contact and are present in saliva and nasal secretions.

3. What is the treatment for this condition?

The treatment for viral throat infections is typically supportive care on the part of the parent. Encourage drinking large amounts of fluids and give medications to control the fever. Bacterial throat infections can be treated with antibiotics.

Some doctors try to prevent sore throats with a low dose of a mild antibiotic for a prolonged time (a preventative treatment known as prophylaxis). There is some concern, however, about using too many antibiotics. The overuse of antibiotics can result in the germs developing a resistance to the drugs, as well as in side effects in children such as allergic reactions. Therefore, prophylaxis is not commonly used.

If a child is very severely affected with recurrent sore throats, particularly if they involve tonsillitis, a doctor may recommend removal of the tonsils and adenoids (the adenoids generally get infected along with the tonsils). Removal of the tonsils and adenoids is referred to as a T&A or tonsillectomy and adenoidectomy.

4. Are there any side effects from the proposed treatment?

The risks of not treating strep throat include spread of the infection to the lymph nodes (glands), blood-borne infections of the joints or bones, infection of the heart muscle, meningitis or other infections in the brain, or infections of the kidneys.

The use of antibiotics to treat bacterial infections may result in side effects in children such as allergic reactions. The overuse of antibiotics may result in the germs developing a resistance to the drugs.

Removing the tonsils and adenoids in a child with recurrent tonsillitis will result in fewer episodes of sore throat. However, removing the tonsils and adenoids cannot prevent anyone from getting a cold or other virus, and occasional illnesses with throat pain may still occur.

The surgery to remove tonsils and adenoids is done under general anesthesia. Modern pediatric anesthesia is extremely safe when given by a trained professional in a well-monitored setting. The most common significant risk of tonsillectomy is bleeding after surgery. When bleeding does occur, it is typically five to ten days after the operation, when the "scab" where the tonsils were falls off. Bleeding that is enough to be noticed happens in about 2 percent to 4 percent of patients, and will be seen as blood in the mouth. Postoperative bleeding from the tonsillectomy site often stops by itself. If bleeding persists it is usually managed by returning to the operating room for a brief procedure under anesthesia to cauterize the bleeding site.

There is also pain after tonsils and adenoids are removed that occasionally is so severe that the child will not be able to drink enough liquid and will become dehydrated. If this happens, the child may require intravenous (IV) fluids. Other risks such as excessive bleeding during surgery, scarring of the throat, and infection are extremely rare.

5. When can my child resume activities?

Your child should be able to resume normal activities when he or she is no longer having a fever and when he or she feels well. Most children are ready to resume normal activity within two or three days.

There is one special area of concern. Children who develop a sore throat related to mononucleosis ("mono") may have associated liver or spleen enlargement. If this occurs your physician may significantly limit their activity level, especially for contact sports, until the enlargement has resolved.

6. How many times does my child need to have this condition before a tonsillectomy is considered?

When a child has recurrent strep throats, does not respond to medical therapy, or does not seem to be "growing out" of the problem, removal of the tonsils and adenoids may be recommended by your physician. There are no universally excepted guidelines for "how many times" a child should have strep throat prior to removal of the tonsils.

There are two factors that your child's physician will consider: the total number of infections and over what duration of time. It is suggested that children with three or more infections of tonsils and/or adenoids per year or enlargement of the tonsil and/or adenoids causing obstruction of the airway during sleep should be considered for removal of the tonsils. A general guideline followed by many physicians is that a child with four or more episodes in six months, six or more episodes in twelve months, or three or more infections per year for several years should be considered for removal of the tonsils and adenoids.

7. If the cause of this condition is strep, do you need to culture other family members and contacts?

When a strep test is positive, many experts recommend treatment or culturing of other family members.

There is a condition known as the "carrier state," in which the child is feeling fine, but a throat culture still shows the presence of the strep bacteria. While this is somewhat controversial, most pediatricians do not treat children who are carriers with antibiotics except in unusual circumstances. They do not seem to be at very high risk for developing heart or kidney damage, and are generally not considered to be very contagious.

8. What precautions need to be observed because of this condition?

Practice good sanitary habits; avoid close physical contact; and avoid sharing of napkins, towels, and utensils with the infected person. Frequent hand washing makes good sense.

See question #2 for additional information.

9. What kind of follow-up is needed?

Generally, in children whose symptoms of strep throat have resolved, no further throat cultures are needed unless the child becomes symptomatic. However, in certain patients that are at an increased risk of complications from strep throat, a repeat culture with treatment of a positive culture may be necessary.

Examples of patients with an increased risk of complications include: those with recurrent symptomatic strep throat in the immediate family or in a closed community; those with a history of rheumatic fever, a known rheumatic fever patient in the family, or known rheumatic fever cases in the community; or those with known heart disease involving the heart valves.

PAUL W. BAUER, MD
Pediatric Otolaryngology

TORSION OF THE TESTICLES

Definition: Twisting of the testicle.

Author's Comment: This condition is considered by some to be a pediatric emergency and, if suspected, warrants immediate diagnosis and treatment.

1. What is the cause of this condition, and how did my child develop it?

Testicular torsion is most commonly seen in males between the ages of twelve and twenty years. Torsion can also occur in newborns. The cause is unknown.

2. What potential problems can develop as a result of this disorder?

When the testicle twists around on its attachment to the body (the spermatic cord), its blood supply becomes compromised. If the blood flow to the testicle is not returned within a matter of hours, the testicle will die. This is an emergency, and boys with testicular pain should be evaluated immediately. Success rates are highest when blood flow is returned to the testicle in less than six hours after the onset of pain.

3. Are there any tests to be done to further define the problem?

If your child has testicular or scrotal pain that is severe in nature, he should be evaluated in an emergency setting. If the diagnosis of testicular torsion is likely, a consultation with the urologist should be obtained without delay. If the diagnosis is less certain, an ultrasound of the testicles performed with Doppler analysis can establish the presence or absence of blood flow to the testicle. Nuclear medicine tests can also be performed to evaluate the testicles. A urinalysis can help to evaluate for urinary tract infection that can sometimes present in a similar fashion if there is involvement of part of the testicle.

4. What can be done to correct the problem?

Prompt surgical exploration and untwisting of the testicle is the treatment for this condition. If the testicle is alive after untwisting, it will be sutured to the inner wall of the scrotum to prevent retorsion (orchiopexy). If the testicle has suffered irreversible damage, it will be removed at the time of surgery. Due to the increased likelihood of torsion on the other side in the future, at the time of exploration most urologists will also perform an orchiopexy on the other testicle.

5. Should we consult a surgeon now?

Yes. The testicle can die if its blood supply is compromised. There are other conditions that may occur in a similar fashion to testicular fashion. These include torsion of an appendix, testis, or epididymis; infection of the testicle or epididymis (epididymoorchitis); or even appendicitis. Depending on the level of suspicion of your physician, a urologist can be consulted immediately or other evaluations (urinalysis, ultrasound, etc.) can be first ordered.

6. Is there a chance that my child will be sterile because of this condition?

The effect of testicular torsion of one testicle on future fertility has not been established. Currently it appears that paternity rates are not effected by torsion on one side. Torsion on both sides is more of a concern as both testicles will have been affected.

7. What can be done to prevent this condition from occurring again?

At the time of repair the affected testicle will be anchored to the wall of the scrotum if it is viable. It will be anchored in such a way to prevent recurrence of the torsion. Also, the other testicle will be similarly fixed to prevent torsion on that side in the future.

8. What kind of follow-up is needed?

Following surgical exploration and fixation of the testicle, reexamination should be performed in six to eight weeks.

WILLIAM STRAND, MD
Urology

UMBILICAL CORD STUMP INFLAMMATION
(Umbilical Granuloma)

Definition: Persistent inflammatory remnant of the umbilical cord located at the base of the belly button.

Author's Comment: This area of raw tissue in the infant's belly button can be easily treated in the office by your child's doctor, with no serious ill effects.

1. What is the cause of this condition, and how did my child develop it?

Umbilical granulomas occur in newborn children as the umbilical cord falls off. They are the result of overgrowth of granulation tissue and can bleed and drain cloudy fluid. Granulation tissue is a normal part of healing and provides a base for skin to grow in over wounds. This tissue grows over spots that need healing, like the belly button after the umbilical cord falls off. An umbilical granuloma occurs when the granulation tissue grows faster than the skin can grow over it and cover the spot. This usually occurs when some form of irritation occurs at the base of the cord or when the umbilical cord stays attached too long.

2. What treatment is needed, or will it heal by itself?

Usually, the only treatment required is to treat the tissue with silver nitrate applied directly to the granuloma (a process called cauterization). This usually kills enough of the granulation tissue so that the skin can grow over the area. Sometimes more than one treatment may be necessary. Rarely, the child may need the area of granulation cut off though this tends to bleed.

3. What are the potential side effects of the treatment?

Occasionally, the silver nitrate can cause mild chemical burns to the surrounding skin around the belly button. Also the silver nitrate can stain the belly button and surrounding skin black, though this usually goes away in about two to three weeks.

4. Will it end up being cosmetically disfiguring in any way?

If the granuloma is completely cauterized (see question #2), the belly button will look normal. Sometimes, skin grows over the granuloma and leaves a small pea-sized bump inside the belly button that will need to be cut out at the family's convenience.

5. Are there any long-term complications from this condition?

Though there are rarely any true complications from umbilical granulomas, there are two disease processes that can mimic umbilical granulomas. A warning sign for these two congenital abnormalities is that silver nitrate treatments do not cure the granuloma, and it will not go away despite local excision.

- Omphalomesenteric remnants: In this condition there is actually a small connection of bowel from the belly button to the intestines. Often green fluid leaks from the belly button that can be foamy and smells bad. This condition can cause the serious problem of intestinal obstruction if the intestines twist around this connection with the belly button.
- Urachal remnants: Patients with this condition have a connection between the belly button and the bladder. Clear fluid (urine) can be noted to drain from the belly button.

Both of these conditions can be differentiated from simple umbilical granulomas by X ray studies as well as sending some of the growth from the belly button to a pathologist for microscopic analysis.

6. Is there any follow-up needed?
Once the granuloma has resolved, no follow-up is necessary.

KEVIN M. KADESKY, MD
Surgery

UMBILICAL HERNIA

Definition: A weakness in the supporting tissues of the umbilicus (navel) permitting the abdominal contents to bulge out.

Author's Comment: The belly-button "outie," as unattractive as it looks, usually resolves on its own over a period of time.

1. What is the cause of this condition, and how did my child develop it?

Newborn infants have a hole in the stiff tissues of the abdominal wall that allows the umbilical cord to pass through. This usually closes on its own after the umbilical cord stump separates. In some children, however, the skin closes properly but there is a weakness left in the stiffer tissues underneath. The "belly button" will then appear to bulge out when the baby cries.

2. What are the potential problems that can occur as a result of this condition?

Very rarely (in less than 1 percent of cases) umbilical hernias can become incarcerated, where the abdominal contents become stuck in the abdominal wall defect. This feels like there is a rock under the skin and it can look reddened and be very tender. This is an emergency and you should contact your doctor immediately.

Some children with umbilical hernias will be teased about its appearance if it is still present when they start school.

3. What will happen if this condition is left untreated?

Most (about 90 percent) will close by themselves by age five. If they are still larger than 1 inch across by age three or are still present at age four, they may have to be repaired. The old folk remedy of taping a coin over the bulge does not work and may be detrimental as it can cause skin irritation and infection.

4. What is the treatment of this condition, and is surgery ever recommended?

We try to repair these prior to the child starting school at age five to six. We may recommend earlier repair for very large hernias.

5. If surgery is needed, when, where, and by whom should the surgery to correct the condition be performed?

The operation should be performed by a pediatric surgeon. It is usually done as day surgery without an overnight stay. Children are kept out of sports or physical education for two weeks after the operation. There are no dietary restrictions.

6. What are the potential complications that can occur as a result of the surgery?

Complications are rare. Some children (especially those whose hernias were very large) will have some additional wrinkled skin at the site after the operation. They generally grow into the stretched skin so it looks more normal with time.

7. When do you wish to see my child again for this condition?

One visit to the surgeon two to three weeks after the operation is usually all that is necessary.

KEVIN M. KADESKY, MD
Surgery

VOMITING

Author's Comment: This condition is a common experience in childhood and can lead to dehydration if it persists. It is wise to contact your child's doctor for information on how to treat the condition and to keep in close communication if the vomiting continues.

1. What is the cause for the vomiting?

Most episodes of vomiting that occur suddenly are caused by a viral infection. This may be associated with fever and/or diarrhea. Other causes for vomiting in childhood include bacterial infections, as well as neurological, kidney, metabolic, and psychological disorders.

2. How long should this condition last, and what problems can occur as a result of it?

The shorter episodes last for up to twenty-four hours, while others may take two to three days to resolve. The main concern is dehydration when the child is unable to keep any fluids down to make up for the losses. Excessive retching from the vomiting may also result in vomiting of blood.

3. Is the condition contagious, and, if so, how is it spread?

Viral causes are contagious. The virus is spread by contamination of the hands or other materials that might enter another person's mouth.

4. What is the treatment for this condition?

There is no medicine for the viral infection. Your pediatrician, however, might prescribe a medication for the nausea or vomiting. The most common ones are Phenergan and Zofran. However, it is important to keep your child adequately hydrated by encouraging him or her to drink small amounts of fluid frequently.

5. If medicines are used, what are their potential side effects?

Most individuals that take Phenergan experience drowsiness within a short time. This usually calms them down and helps them sleep. Some develop dizziness from it.

6. Is any further testing needed to establish the cause for the vomiting?

If the vomiting resolves within a couple of days, no testing is required. If it persists, blood and urine tests may be required. At that time, your doctor may also order special X rays, such as ultrasound, CAT scan, or upper GI series.

7. What symptoms do I look for to determine whether my child is becoming dehydrated?

Dehydrated children usually have decreased urination, dry lips and mouth, and an inability to produce tears when they cry. Drowsiness and lethargy are often signs of severe dehydration.

8. Under what circumstances would I need to call you back?

You need to contact your pediatrician if the vomiting persists beyond a couple of days or if your child complains of headaches, dizziness, blurring of vision, or is unable to walk or is drowsy or lethargic from the onset of the illness. Any concerns regarding dehydration or vomiting of blood should also be brought up promptly with your child's doctor.

9. What kind of follow-up is needed?

If the vomiting completely resolves after a couple of days and your child has returned to normal activity and eating habits, a follow-up with your doctor is not necessary.

ERIC ARGAO, MD
Gastroenterology

Part III
Choosing a Pediatrician

The final weeks for today's expecting parents are filled by making hundreds of decisions. Along with finishing the nursery, arranging maternity leave, and reviewing hospital insurance policies, one very important decision remains—selecting a pediatrician. Choosing a pediatrician is one of the most important decisions you make for your baby's health and future.[1]

Begin your search for a pediatrician at the beginning of pregnancy. Start by asking your friends and relatives who their pediatrician is and if

---

[1] Sylvia Modell, "Choosing a Pediatrician—Based on an Interview with Joel B. Steinberg, MD, Vice President of Medical Affairs and Education at Children's Medical Center of Dallas," *Expectant Mothers Guide to Dallas/Fort Worth* (Pittsburgh, PA: Spindle Publishing Company), 28.

they recommend him or her. Your obstetrician is also a good source to ask. If you're new to an area, check with the county medical society office.[2]

After you've compiled a list of names, arrange for a previsit interview in the pediatrician's office. This is a customary procedure. The visit affords you opportunities, not only to meet the doctor, but also to familiarize yourself with the office waiting room and the general workings of the practice. It is very important that you like what you see, as you will likely be spending a good deal of time here once the baby arrives.

Most interviews do not exceed more than twenty minutes, but it does give you an opportunity to share your concerns and views, so use your time wisely. Be prepared with a list of questions and look for specific qualifications.[3] In doing this, you will be able to get some indication as to how the pediatrician interacts with you and how your personalities and philosophies correlate. Here are some specific questions that you might ask during the interview:*

1. Are you on my health plan, and do you intend to stay on it?
2. How long have you been practicing pediatrics?
3. Are you board certified by the American Board of Pediatrics?
4. Where did you receive your residency training, and have you had any postgraduate training in any subspecialty?
5. Do you have any ongoing relationship with a medical school and, if so, in what capacity?
6. Will you visit my baby in the hospital following delivery, and will the baby be examined every day during its hospital stay?
7. What are your office hours, and are after-hours and weekend visits available?
8. What is the normal wait time in your waiting room?

---

[2] Ibid.

[3] Ibid.

9. Do you schedule checkups and sick visits at separate times during the day, or do you have any other provisions for separating the sick children from the well ones?

10. Under ordinary circumstances, will I see you each visit or will I be rotated to other doctors in the practice or a nurse practitioner?

11. What is your philosophy toward the use of antibiotics in your practice, and do you try to avoid them as much as possible during most minor illnesses?

12. What is the procedure for answering phone calls both during and after office hours, and how long will I usually have to wait for a phone call to be returned? How accessible is the doctor if I would like to speak to him or her?

13. If my child has an emergency after hours or needs to be hospitalized, what hospital(s) do you use?

14. What doctors cover for you when you are not available? Will they have access to my child's records, and are they all on my insurance plan?

15. (If you are choosing a primary care physician who is not a pediatrician) How much training have you had in pediatrics, and what pediatricians do you use for consultation in case of a serious illness?

*The questions listed in this section were specific questions that patients have asked me during interviews through the years. Some of these questions may also be found elsewhere in other printed sources.

Afterword

One of the most prized aspects for me about being a pediatrician is having the privilege of being a trusted advisor to the family. The fact that I can play this role in the lives of people I come in contact with every day is very exciting and continually makes me look forward to being in the office.

I want every parent who comes to my office to leave feeling confident in his or her ability to cope with the illness at hand—indeed, that's why I wrote this book. But I also want every parent to know that babies do not break, and that it's just as important to relax and enjoy your child as it is to teach him or her to crawl or walk or read. Take time for yourself and your spouse. Nap when the baby is napping—it's age-old wisdom, but it's important. Raising kids isn't a sprint—it's a marathon. Pace yourself and enjoy the time you have with them. Eighteen years whizzes by in a flash, and you want to look back and remember that you enjoyed every minute of it. Thank you for letting me be a part of this important process, and HAPPY PARENTING!

—Gary C. Morchower, MD

Index

About the Author

Gary C. Morchower, MD, is a board-certified pediatrician and a Fellow of the American Academy of Pediatrics. He has been in private practice for thirty-seven years and is Clinical Professor of Pediatrics at the University of Texas Southwestern Medical School, where he is very active in the resident teaching program. A graduate of Tulane University and Tulane Medical School, Dr. Morchower has received numerous honors and awards, including the first given Robert L. Moore Outstanding Teaching Award in the field of Pediatrics from Southwestern Medical School. He was recently named recipient of the prestigious 2007 C.D. Taylor Award from Tulane Medical School for distinguished contribution in the field of community medicine.

Dr. Morchower is the past president of the Pediatric Society of Greater Dallas. He has served on numerous boards, including the Dallas Association of Retarded Citizens, the Dallas Chapter of the National Crohn's/Colitis Foundation, and the Dallas Community Council Board to combat childhood obesity.

Dr. Morchower resides in Dallas. He and his wife Bette have been married for thirty years and have two children, Andrew and Karen.

About Medical City
Children's Hospital

Medical City Children's Hospital is a specialty pediatric hospital in Dallas, Texas, exclusively devoted to providing advanced, comprehensive medical care for children and adolescents from birth to age eighteen. Our world-class experience includes helping thousands of children from over seventy-five countries for more than twenty years. As the first hospital in North Texas to achieve the prestigious Magnet designation from the American Nurses Credentialing Center, Medical City Children's Hospital is known for its nursing excellence and expertise in dealing with the unique needs of children and families.

The hospital is home to more than fifty specialty pediatric practices, including nationally and internationally ranked programs in cardiology, congenital heart surgery, craniofacial surgery, hematology/oncology, and emergency medicine. With more than 15,000 procedures completed since 1985, Medical City Children's Hospital's craniofacial program is recognized as one of the leading programs of its kind in the world. More information about Medical City Children's Hospital is available at http://www.mcchildrenshospital.com.